The
A to Z
of Hair, Nails & SKIN

Introduction

This is an extensive revision of the first edition of this book thanks to the many suggestions I have received re inclusions and changes to the book. Most of the pathological terms have been placed in the Common Terms section (CT) which has additional illustrations. This however will not replace *the A to Z of Skin Failure* just as the revised version of ***the A to Z of Bones, Joints, Ligaments & the Back***, did not replace *the A to Z of Bone & Joint Failure*, but rather enhanced it.

The three main sections HAIR, NAILS & SKIN of the Main Text (MT) have remained separate in this edition as in the last, but there is more cross referencing, throughout particularly between the CT section and the MT.

Some Cosmetic procedures are included and summarized as they are in many circles regarded as the normal condition of these tissues, particularly the aging skin.

As always please leave or send FEEDBACK, as it really does make a difference.

The A to Zs may be viewed on 2 sites –
www.amandasatoz.com and
http://www.aspenpharma.com.au/atlas/student.htm

Acknowledgement

Thank you Aspenpharmacare Australia for your ongoing support and assistance in this valuable project.

T0187015

1

Dedication

To all those who have supported me through the tough times.

How to use this book

Think of it and you will find it and if not, **let me know!!**

Try the CT section first particularly for specific terms and then the main text for more general concepts. However not everything can be put into this small volume so you may find it in *the A to Z of Surface Anatomy* or *the A to Z of Endocrinology* or in any of the other *A to Zs*.

Thank you

Amanda Neill
BSc MSc MBBS PhD FACBS

ISBN 978-1-921930-08-9

9 781921 930089

Folklore for
cutting hair & nails

Cut them on Monday,
you cut them for health
Cut them on Tuesday,
you cut them for wealth
Cut them on Wednesday,
you cut them for news
Cut them on Thursday,
a new pair of shoes
Cut them on Friday,
you cut them for sorrow
Cut them on Saturday,
see your true-love tomorrow

Table of contents

HAIR

Development of the Hair Follicle -
Distribution
Growth cycle of the Hair follicle
Loss
Properties
  bonds
  elasticity
  greying / tinting
Regions
Structure of the Hair Follicle - overview
  Bulb
  Cortex & Medulla
  Cuticle
  Shaft
Types - comparisons & overview

Abbreviations

A =	actions / movements of a joint	**Clf =**	chronic inflammation
a =	artery	**CIN =**	carcinoma in situ
aa =	anastomosis (ses)	**CM =**	cell membrane
AA =	alopecia areata	**CN =**	cranial nerve
Ab =	antibody = IL	**CNS =**	central nervous system
Ab/Ag =	antigen antibody complex	**Co =**	collagen
Alf =	acute inflammation	**collat. =**	collateral
AI =	autoimmune	**CP =**	cervical plexus
adj. =	adjective	**CT =**	connective tissue
Ag =	antigen	**D =**	dermis
AKA =	also known as	**Dd =**	deep dermis / reticular dermis
alt. =	alternative	**DD =**	differential diagnosis
ANF =	anti nuclear factor	**DE =**	dermo-epidermal junction
ANS =	autonomic nervous system	**diff. =**	difference(s)
ant. =	anterior	**dist. =**	distal
AR =	allergic reaction	**DLE =**	discoid lupus erythematosus
AS =	Alternative Spelling, generally referring to the diff. b/n UK & USA	**DM =**	Diabetes Mellitus
assoc. =	associated (with)	**Ds =**	desmosome
B =	blood	**DSTL =**	dynamic skin tension lines
B- =	bone marrow derived-	**Du =**	upper dermis / papillary dermis
bc =	because	**Dx =**	diagnosis / diagnoses
BCC =	basal cell carcinoma	**E =**	epidermis
BCR =	B-cell antigen receptor	**EA =**	epidermal appendages
BM =	basement membrane / bone marrow	**EB =**	eyebrow
b/n =	between	**EAM =**	external acoustic meatus
BP =	blood pressure	**EC =**	extracellular (outside the cell)
br =	branch		
BS =	blood supply / blood stream	**e.g. =**	example
BV =	blood vessel	**EL =**	eyelid
Bx =	biopsy	**ER =**	extensor retinaculum
C =	cytoplasm	**Ex =**	examination
CD =	cluster of differentiation	**ext. =**	extensor (as in muscle to extend across a joint)
c.f. =	compared to		

F =	fat / fluid	**jt(s) =**	joints = articulations
Fab =	antibody binding fragment		
		k =	keratotic papule
Fc =	fragment – crystal region	**l =**	lymphatic
		L =	lesion / left
FDP =	follicular dermal papilla / hair papilla	**LL =**	lower limb
		lig =	ligament
FR =	flexor retinaculum	**longit. =**	longitudinal
G =	gland	**LP =**	lamina propria
Ger =	Germany	**Lt. =**	Latin
GF =	growth factors	**m =**	muscle
gld =	gland	**med. =**	medial
GIT =	gastro-intestinal tract	**mem =**	membrane
Gk. =	Greek	**MM =**	mucous membrane
grp =	group	**MNC =**	mononuclear cells
GS =	ground substance	**MO =**	microorganisms
H =	hair	**MT =**	main text
Hb =	haemoglobin	**Mu =**	muscle
HB =	hair bulb	**MV =**	microvilli
HF =	hair follicle	**N (s) =**	nerve(s)
Hg =	haemorrhage	**NA =**	nucleic acids
Histo =	Histology	**NAD =**	normal (size, shape)
HM =	hair matrix	**NAD =**	no abnormality detected
Ho =	hormone		
HS =	hair shaft	**NB =**	nail bed
Hx =	history (of the disease)	**NF =**	nail fold
		NK =	natural killer cells
IAS =	internal anal sphincter	**NM =**	nail matrix
IC =	intracellular	**NMSC =**	non-melanotic skin cancer
If =	inflammation		
IfR =	inflammatory response / reaction	**No =**	nucleolus
		NP =	nail plate
Ig =	mmunoglobulin	**NR =**	nerve root origin
IL =	interleukins = immunoglobulins = Ab	**NS =**	nervous supply / nerve system
Im =	immune	**NT =**	nervous tissue
In =	infection	**Nu =**	nucleus
IR =	immune response / reaction	**nv =**	neurovascular bundle
		P =	pressure / pus
Ix =	investigation of	**PaNS. =**	parasympathetic nervous system
Iy =	injury		

ParaNs = parasympathetic nerves ± fibres
partic = particular(ly)
ph = phalanges
pl. = plural
PMNs = polymorphonuclear cells = polymorphs
PN = peripheral nerve
post. = posterior
proc. = process
prox. = proximal
PSU = pilo-sebacious unit
PVD = peripheral vascular disease
Px = progress / prognosis
R = right / resistance
RBC = red blood cell / enythrocyte
RSTL = relaxed/resting skin tension lines
RT = respiratory tract
S = strata/stratum /sacral
Sb = Stratum basale
Sc = Stratum corneum
SC = spinal cord
SCC = squamous cell carcinoma
sing. = singular
SE = side effects
Sg = Stratum granulosum
SL = Stratum lucidum
SLE = systemic lupus erythematosus
Sm = Stratum malphigii
SN = spinal nerve
SP = spinous process / sacral plexus
SPF = sun protection factor
Ss = Stratum spinosum
SS = signs and symptoms
STL = skin tension lines

Su = subcutaneous T / fat
subcut. = subcutaneous (just under the skin) as a site
supf = superficial
SyNS = sympathetic nervous system
T = tissue
TJC = tight junctional complex
Tm = Tumour
TNF = tumour necrosis factor
Tx = treatment / therapy
UL = upper limb, arm
v = vein
V = vertebra
VB = vertebral body
VC = vertebral column
VDRL = Venereal Disease Research Laboratory (test for syphilis)
vv = visa versa
w = with
WBCs = white blood cells / leucocytes
w/n = within
w/o = without
wrt = with respect to
ZA = Zonular adherens
ZO = Zonular occudens
& = and
∩ = intersection with

A to Z of terms & definitions

descriptions of skin conditions & lesions – including physiological &/or pathological changes *

general, anatomical & pathological terms

immunological, inflammatory terms

prefixes / suffixes

The pronunciation guide to words in this section are in bold green lettering

Stressed syllables are in CAPITAL LETTERS

Vowel sounds are pronounced as indicated below

A	May	ay
	map	a
	mark	ah
E	Me	ee
	met	e
	term	ur
I	eye / sight	ï
	tin	i
O	go	oh
	mother	uh
	mop	o
	more	or
	boy	oi
	lose	oo
	nook	oe
	loose	ou
U	blue	oo
	cute	ew
	cut	uh
Y	family	ee
	myth	i
	eye	ï

*note there is often an overlap with these terms in that case if the term is mainly used to denote skin features this colour will take precedence

ABCDE

system to describe skin changes

and detect neoplasia - melanoma

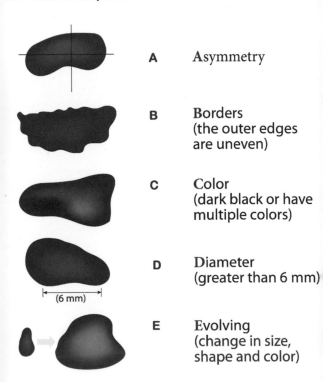

A Asymmetry

B Borders
(the outer edges
are uneven)

C Color
(dark black or have
multiple colors)

D Diameter
(greater than 6 mm)

(6 mm)

E Evolving
(change in size,
shape and color)

Abscess (AB-ses) *Lt ab = away cedere = to go = to go away*
a localized circumscribed collection of pus buried in a cavity of
necrotic tissue in the skin at any level (& other organs)

  Aetiology In, ± Staph aureus

  Histo – localized collection of PMNs
when other inflammatory cells are included = suppuration
abcesses + Hf = furuncle
see also **Boil, Empyema, Furuncle, Phlegmon, Suppuration**

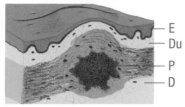

acantho- (AY-kan- thoh) **relating to spine or thorn**

Acantholysis *Gk thorn prickle loosening of*

breakdown of cell to cell junctions in epithelial cells due to deterioration
of ic cement - which may collapse in a blister / cleft

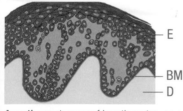

Aetiology - AI
Histo - loosening of the Ds
found at the levels of the
prickle cells, granular cells
± basal layers

Acanthoma tumour of keratinocytes, as squamous epithelial cells

Acanthosis *Gk thorn, prickles*

thickened skin - diffuse hyperplasia of the SMalpighii (ie SGranulosum
+ SSpinosum)

  Aetiology - autoimmune

  Histo - increased spinocytes /granulocytes & cornified layer

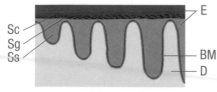

Acanthosis nigricans a diffuse, asymptomatic, symmetric, velvety thickening & darkening of the skin, chiefly in the armpits & other body folds & MMs. The skin appears dirty & thick in the areas of involvement. **DD adenocarcinoma.**

Acid mantle the various factors on the skin which cause it to have an acid pH. The major contributor of this is sebum, *see also* **pH scale.**

Acne (AK-nee) *Gk acme = point / chaff* represents a number of conditions resulting from blockage of the pilo-sebaceous unit with debris Di &/or keratin ± If, ± In – Acne is the result of a single process but presents in a number of different ways depending upon the severity & extent of the acne process & blockage(s) and spread of the In. It is found in the facial, cervical & back regions. The commonest type is **acne vulgaris**, appearing before puberty & continuing > 30yo. *see also* **Comedoe, Pustule, Sycosis**

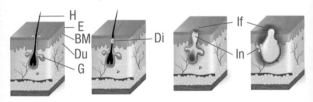

Baby Acne is a general term to describe 3 different types of acne in newborns & infants.

1. **neonatal milia** - multiple tiny whiteheads on the face of newborns, occurs in half of all newborns – is self limiting
2. **neonatal acne** appears after birth – typical pustules looks more like teenage acne, not as severe - typically resolves after a few months.
3. **Infantile acne** occurs at 3-4 months looks like regular acne with blackheads, whitehead, pimples and pustules. It may last 2 to 3 years, familial seen in boys only due to maternal androgens .
4. **Acne Excoriee** acne with excoriations as features on the sites due to the patient scratching away the comedones & creating "sores"
5. **Acne Keloides** nodules developing in Keloid or scar tissue
6. **Acne Necrotica** presents in adult men as itchy painful papules and pustules which leave scars and hair loss, possibly due to an In but not related to "**Acne Vulgaris**"

acro- (adj acral) Gk akcron = extreme end, extremity, peak, tip, denoting something at the extremities ankles / wrists

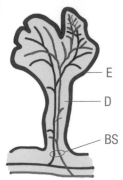

Acrochodon (AK-roh-kord-on) AKA Fibroepithelial polyp AKA Skin Tag small, growths of skin that individuals develop around the eyelids, neck, armpits, & the groin. They appear as small little balls of skin attached to the body by a thin stalk. They are benign & familial; predisposing factors are obesity & frictional P on the skin. They increase with age, most people > 40yo will have at least one. *see also* **Polyp**

Actinic (AK-tin-ik) referring to the light rays over and above the UV and which can cause skin damage **AKA Solar.**

Actinic keratoses *see* **Keratosis**

Adaptability wrt afferent skin N receptors – when stimulated in a long constant manner, N adapt i.e. they return to their normal firing rate either quickly "phasic" Ns e.g. when putting on clothes they rapidly become "undetected" or slowly "tonic" Ns, e.g. when balancing the position is constantly reported.

Adaptive immunity = Adaptive IR = Aquired IR the response of Ag-specific lymphocytes to Ab, including the development of immunologic memory. Adaptive IRs are distinct from the innate & non-adaptive phases of immunity, which are not mediated by clonal selection of Ag-specific lymphocytes. *See also* **Immunity**

Additus opening /entrance

adeno-(a-den-OH) gland

Adenoid (ad-EN-oyd) gland

Adenoma benign glandular tumour e.g. sebaceous adenoma in skin - 2-4mm to 1cm yellowish cyst with sebum discharge *see also* **sebaceous cyst**

Adipocytic metaplasia - changing of the tissue to fat like cells

Adiposis Dolorosa AKA Dercum's disease painful plaques of bruised hardened fat
Aetiology - idiopathic

Adnexa(e) (AD-nex-uh / AD-nex-ee) appendices or adjunct parts e.g. in the skin, the glands, hair & nails are also derived from the epidermal layer: additional structures pertaining to the main structure; extras

Age Spots *see* **Keratosis, Lentigo** - this general term indicates a large range of brown marks on the skin which increase in numbers & size with age. They differ from freckles in that they are larger ↑ with age, may be raised on the skin, appear mainly on the hands, feet and face and rarely on other areas even with sun exposure. They are a sign of epidermal breakdown

Albinism complete lack of melanin formation of the skin and eyes - white skin and hair pale iris - poor eyesight and extreme photosensitivity

Albright's syndrome syndrome of polyostotic fibrous dysplasia of bones – and precocious puberty with large café-au-lait lesions up to 10cm *see also* **Café-au Lait patches**

Allergic reaction (AR) an abnormally high reaction of the Im system to specific substances, e.g. pollens, foods or MOs. Common sites of the AR include the skin & MM (including the GIT & RT).

Allergic Contact Dermatitis *see* **Dermatitis**

Alopecia (al-OH-peesh- uh). **AKA Baldness** hair loss

Alopecia areata well defined round patches of hair loss all over the scalp which may become generalized - areas are bordered by **Exclamation point hairs**

    Alopecia areata monolocularis: a single bald spot on the scalp. **AAM**

    Alopecia areata multilocularis: multiple bald spot on the scalp. **AAMx**

    Alopecia areata totalis: loss of all the hair on the scalp. **AAT**

    Alopecia areata universalis: all body hair, + pubic hair, is lost. **AAU**

    Alopecia areata barbae: loss is only in the beard region, usually patchy. **AAB**

    AAM   AAMx   AAT   AAU   AAb

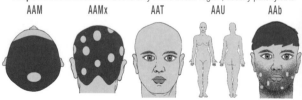

Androgenetic alopecia = male pattern alopecia AM hair miniaturization and loss due to the presence of androgens, beginning at the vertex and forehead there is diffuse hair loss & thinning which variably extends to become complete in these areas – there may be sparring of the temporal & occipital areas.

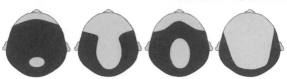

= **female pattern alopecia AF** similar to male pattern except that there is seldom frontal loss & the loss is more diffuse a thinning rather than balding. *See also* **Hair loss**

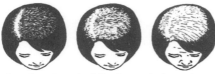

Scarring alopecia defined areas in the scalp causing hair follicle destruction and permanent hair loss associated with **Discoid Lupus, Lichen plano pilaris**.

Tension alopecia AKA traction alopecia AT: hair loss develops along the frontal margins & temporal margins of the scalp due to constant tension on the hair from being tied very tightly – or pulled harshly in styling – Temporal area is particularly suspectible as the hair here is generally thinner. *See also* **Hair loss**

Alveolus air filled eg. bone - tooth socket *adj - alveolar* (as in air filled bone in the maxilla)

Anagen 1st stage of hair cycle - synthesis of the hair

Anaesthesia loss of sensation

Androgenetic alopecia *see* **Alopecia**

angio (anj-EE-oh) – to do with BVs

Angioectasias AKA Telangeclasia

Angioedema swelling of tissues due to engorgement & permeability of the BVs & hence the surrounding Ts most affected are MM including the MMs of the GIT & RT part of lf

Angioma (anj-EE-oh-mah) - tumour of BVs which are dilated and expanded, it may involve other organs as well as the skin.

On the skin they all blanch when pressed and then "refill' with B with the release of P

Cherry Angioma AKA Senile angioma smooth round dome elevated bright pink, multiple, familial, in numbers with age- bleeds only

Port Wine birthmark, Sturge-Weber syndrome, presents as a dark red / purple pigmented well demarcated lesion may be quite extensive & involve other tissues

Capillary Angioma AKA Salmon patch presents as a pink mark on the occiput of the head or face & may resolve

Lymphangiomas tumour of the lymphatics

Spider Angiomas present as a network of capillaries on the skin with a central enlarged spot and "legs" coming out -
DD Telangectasia

Angiolymphoid hyperplasia AKA Kimura' disease acquired eruption of small ill-defined violacious subcut. nodules in the head & neck region

Angiosome a region from the skin to the one supplied by the one source BV

Anhydrosis AS Anhidrosis, AKA Adiaphoresis AKA Sweating deficiency total or partial failure of sweat glands - as opposed to **Hyperhydrosis**

Aetiology due to reduced SyNS *see also* **Eccrine glands, Dyshydrosis, Hypohydrosis**

Anlagen *Ger the laying down of* - in embryonic terms the group of cells which cluster together and later form specialized structures

Annular descriptive term to mean concentric circles *see also* **Target lesions**

Anogen active growth phase of the hair

Ansa - a loop like structure

Anthrax In caused by *Bacillus anthracis*, in both animals and man. The spore can exist dormant for decades. It is v contagious.

Skin presentation - a tender red pustule on the skin which becomes a **malignant pustule**, with an hemorrhagic crust, & small vesicopustules surrounding the central lesion, fever, malaise & death can occur w/n a week.

anti- against

Antibodies (Abs) self molecules which are synthesized by the Im cells after being exposed to Ags. *See also* **Immunoglobulin**

Antigen (Ag) usually a foreign macromolecule that triggers the IR and the production of Abs and other immune active molecules e.g. **tumor necrosis factor (TNF)**. *adj antigenic*

Antigen – presenting cells *see* **Dendritic cells.**

Anti-inflammatory anything which ↓ inflammation by acting on body responses not the causative agent(s).

Aperture an opening or space b/n bones or w/n a bone.

Aphtha *pl aphthae adj aphthous / aphthoid Gk ulceration* small ulcer with a grey centre & red halo generally on the MM.

Aphthous (AFF-thus) ulcers *Gk aphtha = ulcer* AKA **Canker sores** recurrent oral ulcers of unknown aetiology, present as white plaques in the mouth & lips common in immunodepressed &/or susceptible patients

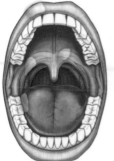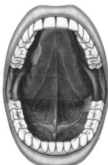

Aplasia lack of cell growth *Lt a = w/o plasia = growth*

apo- away from / detached

Apocrine (ap-OH-krin) glands a type of gland where the apical region is sloughed off along (mercrine or decapitation secretion) with its secretions - e.g. apocrine sweat glands are in the axilla & groin regions they are the **Scent sweat glands** (surrounded by myoepithelial cells (Me) to assist in contraction & attached to genital hairs) as opposed to the **Eccrine sweat glands** – *see also* **Holocrine**

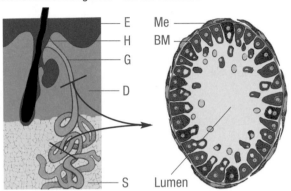

See also **SKIN – epidermis appendages**

Apocrine hidrocystoma - tumour of apocrine glands often resulting in excess smelly sweat blockage of the Apocrine glands resulting in smelly groins and armpits = Fox-Fordyce disease

Apoptysis *Gk aptos = to drop out*
pockets of dead or dying cells in normal healthy tissue - programmed cell death - found at the levels of the skin and in all organs
Aetiology – anoxia
Histo – individual cell death in healthy cells

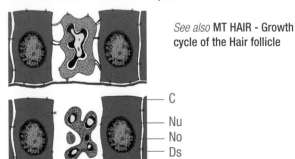

See also **MT HAIR - Growth cycle of the Hair follicle**

© A. L. Neill

Appendicular refers to the appendices of the axial i.e. in the skeleton, the arms & legs which hang from the axial skeleton, this also includes the pectoral and pelvic girdles (not the Sacrum)

Arbor *Gk treelike branches – adj. arborizing,* branching

Areata (ARY-ar-tar) patches / occurring in patchy distribution

Argyria exposure to silver skin & nails show blue-black diffuse colouration

Astringent a shrinking agent, a solution which shrinks body tissues &/or organs. It may also have drying properties.

Athlete's foot AKA Tinea Pedis a fungal In of the feet, presentation itchy scaly rash on the soles and b/n the toes with cracks and fissures in extreme cases. Closed shoes and sweaty feet are predisposing factors

Atopy (AY-top-ee) *Gk atopis = out of place* group of diseases characterized by the tendency to have a severe hypersensitive reaction to common materials as in the RT GIT and skin *adj atopy = allergic* as in *atopic dermatitis* = skin If responding to contact with a substance over-stimulating the IR -

Atrophy (a-TROH-fee) *Gk a = lack of, trophe = nourishment* deterioration of T or organ wrt skin loss of thickness or substance of the skin &/or one of its components – thinner, frailer skin -

　epidermis = lichen sclerosis
　dermis = focal dermal hypoplasia
　elastic tissue atrophy = anetoderma
　&/or subcutaneous fat = lipoatrophy

This may be a normal process with aging where the skin becomes weaker, and more translucent with loss of collagen fibres & epithelial thickness, subject to tearing and poor healing.

　Histo - smaller fewer cells ± extracell material & fibres in one or more of the skin layers

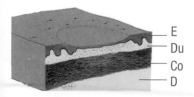

E
Du
Co
D

Atypical not normal, unusual presentation of a phenomenon or structure

auto- self

Autoimmune (Aim) pertaining to cells & Abs that arise from & are directed against the individual's own tissues i.e. against "self"

Axilla = armpit pertaining to the triangular region at the top of the UL & the upper thoracic wall – the underarm

Axis *adj axial* refers to the head & trunk (vertebrae, ribs & sternum) of the body – not arms or legs

B cells = B lymphocytes 1 of the 2 major types of lymphocyte. B means the cells come originally from the BM *see also* **Plasma cells, T cells, WBCs.**

"Baby acne" *see* **Acne**

Baldness *see* **Alopecia, HAIR – Hair loss**

Ballooning development of air pockets in the epidermal layer of the skin

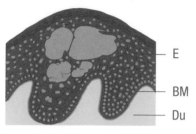

- E
- BM
- Du

Balanitis *Gk balano = penis* If of the glans penis *see also* **Phimosis**

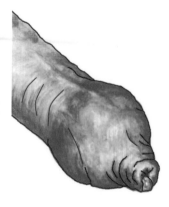

Barbae Beard

Barlow's disease – Scurvy in infants *see* **Scurvy**

Basal bottom - in skin and the GIT & RT - this is the layer which divides and supplies cells for the other epithelial layers

Basal cell carcinoma (BCC) cancer of the basal epithelial cells **(Sb)**. Well demarcated translucent nodules ± telangectasia ± pigmentation with rounded edges ± central ulceration

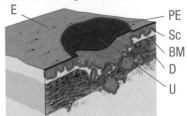

Morpheic BCC = Sclerosing BCC presents as an expanding white plaque on the skin's surface

Sites: face & areas of cartilage/skin fusion e.g. the ears, nose, also in sun-exposed areas & corners of the eyes. Although neoplastic BCCs do not metastasize as they don't invade through their BM

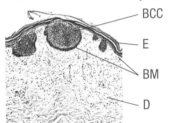

Rodent BCC highly invasive BCC found on the face near nose - invades along ducts eg lacrimal duct destroying nasal tissue. May present as a blocked tear duct

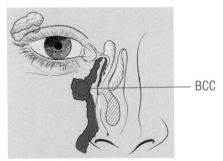

Basement Membrane (BM) protein fibrillar matrix upon which all the base epidermal layers rest – barrier b/n the epidermis & dermis and in MMs the epidermal lining and the mucosa below. Consists of 2 layers Lamina lucida - connecting the epithelial cells and Lamina densa - a fibrillar layer facing the dermis. *See also* **SKIN - Dermis**

baso- base as in acid / base and in the bottom – the basal layer

Basophils - granulocytes of the Im system which take up base staining because of high acid cytoplasmic granules *see also* **Acidophils, Neutrophils & PMNs, WBCs.**

Beau's lines lines or grooves across the nail caused by traumatic factors e.g. shock *see* **MT - NAILS - Abnormal Nail Shape**

Becker's Naevus *see* **Naevus**

Bed Bugs AKA Wall louse AKA Mahogany flat AKA Chinche bug AKA Redcoat = insects of the CIMEX genus – common bed bug = Cimex lectularius are parasitic insects 4-5 X 2-3 mm which feed on human blood. Although commonly found in bedding and feeding nocturnally; they may be active in the day and found wherever humans collect. They can survive for up to a year w/o feeding but generally feed every 5-10 days.

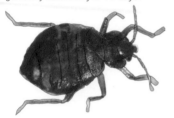

Bed bug bites = Cimicosis present as blisters to rashes - may lead to a range of skin manifestations from no visible effects to prominent blisters and erythematous rash. In some patients they may have a psychological effect. They do not infect humans with any pathogens but may carry up to 28.

Bed sores *see* **Decubitus ulcers**

Behçert's disease immune related systemic vasculitis which present as aphthous ulcers on the MM of the GIT, genital areas, RT & eyes. This disease can be Dx by eliciting pathergy, and is generally accompanied by GIT symptoms **DD Pyoderma Gangrenosum** *see also* **Pathergy**

Benign a cellular / tissue growth which is not controlled by normal factors but which does not metastasize. It may invade other organs or tissues and recur if removed but it will not break off and spread to other areas, as opposed to malignant.

Benign Familial Chronic Pemphigus = Hailey-Hailey disease a reduction in the number of Ds of the skin – increasing the epithelial fragility. It appears as thin walled blisters in the skin fold areas – axilla, groin & neck groin that easily rupture into erosions. **DD Keratosis Follicularis = Darier's disease**

> **Benign Mucosal Pemphigus = Cicartrical Pemphigus** blistering disorder on the MM which leaves permanent scarring *see also* **Pemphigus**

Beri Beri disease due to Thiamine deficiency

Biopsy (Bx) section of a T /organ is taken to Dx the condition generally at right angles to the T surface – e.g. skin Bx small piece of the affected skin is removed around the lesion with a little disturbance of the area as possible

> **Punch Bx** – a cone of T is taken containing all the skin layers. The T should be disturbed as little as possible so the microanatomy is not distorted

good technique   *poor technique*

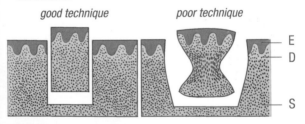

— E
— D

— S

Shave Biopsy – only in the skin – removing T by slicing along the layers – maybe only to gather epidermis

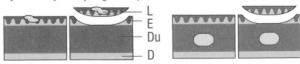

— L
— E
— Du
— D

– not suitable for deeper lesions as it may miss the lesion

see also **Curette, Micrographic surgery AKA Moh's technique**

     © A. L. Neill

Birefringent used to describe crystals which split light waves into two unequally reflected or transmitted waves – seen in some skin crystalline deposits

Birth mark is any congenital defect of the skin so it may refer to a number of deformities although it usually refers to **Epidermal Naevus** *see also* **Naevus**

Black Heel = Talon noir sudden pigmentation on the heel caused by trauma – seen on runners, blood has escaped into the epidermis & resolves spontaneously **DD Melanoma**

Blackhead *see* **Comedo**

Blanchable a mark on the skin which can be whitened when the area is pressed and re-colours when the P is released i.e. the B is still in BVs and not in the T so may be "squeezed" away to return with release. ≠ **Purpura, non blanchable**

> **Glass test** - common test for this is to place a glass on the skin & push
> +ve - if the skin goes pale through the glass
> –ve - if the skin stays red through the glass

Blashko's lines = Cutaneous Mosaicsm lines present in the skin on the back in a large V-shape, following the embryological migration pathway – they represent 2 distinct dermal populations present side by side in the one person. Normally invisible they are enhanced with other diseases such as **chimera, focal dermal hyperplasia, sebaceous naevus & Shingles** *see also* **Koebner phenomenon**

-blast immature cell / undifferentiated cell

blepho- pertaining to the eyelid

Blister a fluid filled sac *see also* **Bullae, Vesicle**

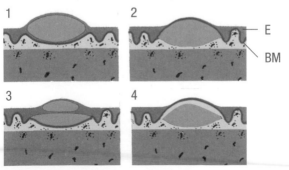

It may be located – in the epidermis – intra-epidermal 1
under the epidermis – subepidermal 2
both in & under the epidermis 3
and in the dermis 4

Blood Blister *see* **Haematoma**

Blue Naevus *see* **Naevus**

Blushing AKA Flushing

Boggy – soft wet swelling as used to describe ringworm lesions

Boil *see* **Furuncle**

BO-TOX a trademark for a preparation of botulinum toxin produced by bacterium ***Clostridium botulinum***, used to treat muscle spasm of all kinds: blepharospasms, strabismus, and muscle dystonias.

A well known SE is to smooth facial wrinkles.

Aetiology - the bacterial toxin (Bot) blocks the neurotransmitter, Acetylcholine (Ach) from connecting the nerve to the muscle (Mu) & so the muscle cannot contract – & the overlying skin will not wrinkle

NEUROMUSCULAR JUNCTION –

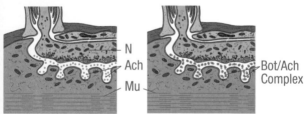

N
Ach
Mu
Bot/Ach Complex

Boss a smooth round broad eminence - mainly in the frontal bone female > male

Bowen's disease = squamous CIN AKA Keratoacanthoma an intraepidermal neoplastic disease on the skin of the LL (although may be anywhere) presenting as an irregular spreading erythematosus plaque, with surface crusting &/or scaling *see also* **Erythroplasia of Queyrat, SCC**

Breslow thickness levels measure used to describe the Px and survival rate of melanoma, in conjunction with other indicators e.g. the Clark's levels and histopathological descriptions. The maximum thickness of the melanoma after surgical removal is measured and then tabulated as follows:

- less than 1 mm: 5-year survival is 95% to 100%
- 1 to 2 mm: 5-year survival is 80% to 96%
- 2.1 to 4 mm: 5-year survival is 60% to 75%
- greater than 4 mm: 5-year survival is 37% to 50%

Bromhidrosis particularly pungent sweat due to secretions of the apocrine sweat glands generally due to bacterial Ins but may be due to diet

Bruise *see* **Haematoma**

Buccal *Lt bucca = cheek* pertaining to the cheek *see also* **Malar**

Bulla (BULL-uh) *pl Bullae Lt bulla = bubble* large fluid-filled unlined space w/n the epidermis or epidermo-dermal junction interchangeable with Vesicle although bulla tends to indicate a bigger structure > 5mm *see also* **Blister, Vesicle**

Bullous = Pemphigoid adj to describe an disease to the BM of the epithelium in the elderly, presents as red blistering patches either local or widespread which may be denuded & so allow for 2° Ins to develop.

Bunion *Gk bounion = turnip* abnormal prominence on the inner aspect of the 1st MT head + a bursa & valgus (lat) displacement of the Hallux (big toe)

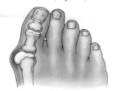

Bunionette AKA Taylor's bunion enlargement of the lat aspect of the 5th MT head

Burrow = Cuniculus tunnel in the skin – generally the epidermis caused by an MO or parasite *see also* **Scabies**

Bursa a saclike cavity filled with viscid fluid caused by friction to alleviate tissue trauma – may occur at several levels generally b/n layers ie b/n epidermis /dermis – dermis / fascial layer – etc. *see also* **Blister**

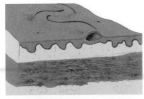

Café-au lait patch / plaque defined coffee coloured area on the skin indicative of more serious systemic disease particularly if multiple spots are present *see also* **Albright's disease, Neurofibromatosis, Plaque**

Calcinosis (KAL-sin-oh-sis) deposits of Calcium in body tissues &/or organs

Calculus (KAL-que-lus) mineral deposit in tissue *see also* **stone**

Callus (KAL-us) localized hyperplasia of the SCorneum due to friction *see also* **Bunion, Hyperkeratosis, Keratoma**

Calor heat – 1 of the cardinal signs of If *see also* **Inflammation**

Calvaria refers to the cranium w/o the facial bones attached as opposed to the **Splanchnocranium** – the facial bones of the skull.

Campell de Morgan spots *see* **Cherry Angioma, Angioma**

Canal *adj canular* = tunnel / extended foramen as in the carotid canal at the base of the skull (canicular - small canal)

Candida (KAN-dee-dar) yeast-like fungi - some species are normal flora others result in infections on the skin & MMs eg the vaginal wall.

Cancer = Neoplasia an uncontrolled growth of cells

Canities (KARH-nish-eez) the amount of "whiteness" or greyness in the hair **AKA Poliosis, Poliothrix**

Capillary (KAP-il-er-ee) *Lt hair-like* small BVs, which consist of endothelium lying on BM. No muscle layer or adventitia in the BVs

Capillary Angioma AKA Salmon patch - presents as a pink blanchable patch usually on the face (A). If present from birth may fade in childhood. Caused by cavernous malformation of the dermal capillaries, which can be seen through the epidermis *see also* **Angioma DD Port wine stain**

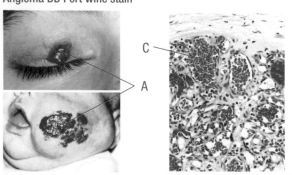

Carbuncle (KAR-bung-kl) *Gk carbunculus = little coal* large furuncle with multiple heads, necrotizing In of the skin & subcut. T causing severe localized Alf.

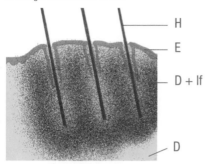

-**carcinoma (KAR-sin-oh-mah)** cancer of epithelial cells

Carcinoma in situ (CIN) cancerous focal changes in the epithelium, above the BM. One of the changes seen is a change in the TJC so that the epithelial cells do not adhere to each other as usual.

Cell The smallest unit of living structure capable of independent existence, composed of a membrane-enclosed mass of protoplasm containing a nucleus or nucleoid material.

Cellulite = *"cottage cheese skin"* Skin develops a dimpling/puckering (like orange peel) effect - due to fat cells swelling in the subcutaneous T **(F)**. Fibrous septa of collagen **(Co)** connecting the dermis with the underlying deep fascia become stretched due to the expanded fat globules. Globules may contain fats + other substances which draw in fluids and so increase their size. This may end up compromising the BS

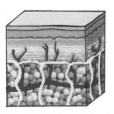 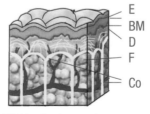

of the skin by "squashing the BVs" leading to necrosis.

Cellulitis If of the cells in the deep subcut. T, generally due to bacterial In Staph or Strep – widespread – as opposed to Abscess which is localized *see also* **Phlegmon**

29

-centric (SEN-trik) central / with a centre

Cephalic (KEF-al-ik) pertaining to the head

cerat AS **kerat** corney, hard horney tissue

cervico- (SERV-i-coh) pertaining to the neck

Chancre *adj –chancoid Lt cancer = crab* destructive sore usually the primary painless lesion of syphilis but also the cutaneous site of inoculation &/or In

Cheloid *see* **Keloid (KEE-loyd)**

cheil- (KĪ-I) AKA chil- pertaining to lips

Cheilitis (KEE-lĭ-tis) If of the lips *see also* **Perlèche**

Cheilosis AKA Cracked lips non-If cracking of the lips often assoc. with abnormalities of the upper GIT

chemo- (KEE-moh) chemically induced

Chemokines substances which stimulate the activation, division & migration of cells, generally leucocytes *see also* **Leucokines.**

Chemotaxis a directed movement of cells due to their reaction of released chemical substances

Cherry Angiomas AKA Senile Angiomas present as smooth bright red "moles" - but they are blanchable. They are one of the most common growths that occur on the skin, increasing in number with age.

They are malformations of the capillaries; if knocked they can bleed profusely *see also* **Angiomas, Polyps.**

Chicken Pox *see* **Herpes Zoster, Varicella**

Chilblains recurrent localized redness & doughy subcut. swelling (like potatoes) on the digits & facial extremities due to cold exposure accompanied by pain & itching – *see also* **Perniosis**

Chimera (KIM-er-uh) = *Gk Chimera – mythical beast made up from various animals* with an organism which possess 2 or more origins as in a person with an organ transplant – or congenitally someone with 2 sets of DNA *see also* **Mosaic**

Chloasma (KLOH-az-muh) hyper-pigmented skin *see* **Melasma**

Cholinergic (KOL-in-er-jik) = Parasympathomimetic symptoms due to the overstimulation of the PaNS

chondro- (KON-droh) referring to cartilage

Chondordermatitis AKA Winkler's disease referring to the If on the helix of the ears, painful non-contagious appears >30yrs

chromo- referring to colour

Cicatrix (sik-AH-triks) *adj cicatricial* (sik-AH-trish-al) = scar tissue derived from granulomae

Cimicosis (simi-KOH-sis) *see* **Bed Bugs**

Circinate annular or circular

Clavus *see* **Bunions, Corns**

Clark's naevus *see* **Dysplastic naevis = abnormal mole** *see* **Naevus**

Clark levels levels used to describe the extent of spread of a melanoma

I   confined to the epidermis
II invasion of the papillary (upper) Dermis
III present in the upper dermis but NOT in the lower
IV penetration to the reticular (lower) Dermis
V penetration to the subcutaneous fat

and so to predict the outcome of Tx – used in conjunction with histopathological tissue description – and Breslow levels
see also **Breslow levels**

Clavus *pl Clavi see* **Bunions, Corns**

Cleanser a cleaning agent – in skin used to remove debris, oil, dead skin cells.

Complications with application

> **1 pH changes**, generally soap has a pH of 9-10 & the skin pH is ~ 5.5 so excessive use can alter the pH of the normal skin bacterial flora – geophytes
>
> **2 excessive removal of skin oils** – excessive removal of sebum will cause the sebaceous glands to ↑ their production of sebum; this could lead to blocked pores, acne & the development of oily skin
>
> **3 allergic reaction** – components of the cleanser can cause IR & the sensitizing of the skin
>
> **4 drying of the skin** – dissolving of the oily keratin of the SCorneum can result in dry skin & the complications – so moisturizers are often usd in conjunction with cleansers
>
> *see also* **Moisturizers**

Cleft separation of the top epithelial layers and those of the basal layers may occur at any stratum – This is a suprabasal cleft.

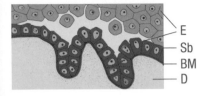

E
Sb
BM
D

Clones series of cells which are identical to each other; in the IR these are lymphocytes which all produce the same Ags &/or cytokines

Clubbing AKA Hippocratic fingers AKA Drumstick fingers a proliferation of subcut. Ts in the terminal phalanges w/o osseous changes. Normal Lovibond (finger/nail) angle 160° increases to >180°

Aetiology thoracic diseases (Heart &/or Lungs) generalized chronic hypoxia, idiopathic *see also* **NAILS Nail Plate shape abnormalities**

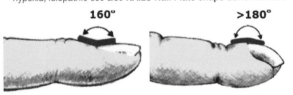

160°   **>180°**

Clusters descriptive term for multiple cells seen to be together but not orientated in any particular manner as opposed to nests

Clusters of differentiation (CD) immune cells which express glycoproteins on their surfaces and are seen to act together – specific molecules may be referred to as numbers as in CD4 cells (used to be called leu-3)

Clusters of PMNs used to indicate areas of Alf filled with PMNs (neutrophils which have left the BS)

Cold Sores *see* **Herpes**

Collarette a narrow rim of loosened keratin overhanging the periphery of a circumscribed skin lesion, attached to the normal surrounding skin.

Comedo AKA Blackhead AKA Whitehead *pl comedone / comedones (note the plural is often used as a singular term in the literature)* **(KOM-e-dohn)** a non-If lesion of acne consisting of a sebum or keratin plug around the dilated hair follicle orifice ± bacterial In *see also* **Epithelial cysts**

Open Comedo AKA Blackhead (lesion is exposed to air & dirt)

Closed Comedo AKA Whitehead (lesion is covered by epithelium and avascular)

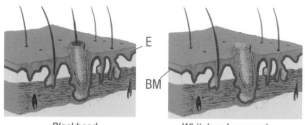

Blackhead
open follicle

Whitehead covered
blocked follicle

Complement *Lt to fill up or fill out* an entire protein cascade in the BS activated by the presence of BM &/or necrotic cell components, may also be activate din the tissues by allogens – allergic Ag

Complex in IR the combining of 2 factors involved in the IfR or the IR e.g. an Ag & Ab complex which combines to activate or further develop the inflammatory process.

Concha (KONG- ku) *pl.* **conchae** (KONG- kee) *adj. chonchoid* a shell shaped bone as in the ear or nose old term for Turbinate.

Condyloma (KON-dee-loh-muh) *Gk knuckle / knob or wart* CT core with an epithelial covering & papilloma structure

Condyloma Acuminata a venereal wart(s) grow in the genital regions – vulva & penis). Considered a very common STD. Highly contagious and multiple, it can occur at any age, but most frequently in adults. Aetiology the Human papilloma virus, HPV which infects the skin. It is considered to be precancerous.

Congenital - existing at birth.

Corn *see also* **Bunion, Callus, Clavus** horny outgrowth of the foot – localized hyperplasia of the SCorneum - in response to excessive friction sometimes due to ill-fitting shoes &/or loss of protective fat pads in the foot with age

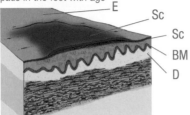

Corneocytes outer layer in HS cuticle of curved keratinocytes also in the skin important in preserving the moisture content of the hair & skin and devoid of any IC structures except keratin

Corona *adj.- coronary, coronoid or coronal* a crown, hence a coronal plane is parallel to the main arch of a crown which passes from ear to ear (c.f. coronal suture).

Corp *adj corporis* body (of anything) similar to Trunk / Torso

Corpuscle (KOR-pus-I) *Lt corpusculum = little body* in blood refers to an unattached body cell such as a blood or lymph cell
in skin this refers to a rounded globular mass of cells as attached to pressure receptors in the skin

Cortex the rind or the bark of the tree

Cracked lips *see* **Cheilosis**

Cradle cap *see* **Dermatitis**

Creases AKA skin creases AKA perma lines AKA wrinkles *see* **Wrinkles**

-crine (KRINE) secreting

Crown = Vertex the top of the organ or body – **re hair** this refers to the site on the scalp where the hair growth centers and grows from in all directions – the site where male pattern baldness commences

Crura *adj cruris* leg

Crust AKA Scab usually a dry serum exudates (serous crust) – or a thick mass of horny cells (keratin crust) or a mixture of both

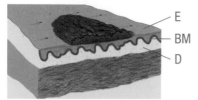

Cuniculus *see* **Burrow**

Curette AKA Curet *Fr cureter to scrape* an instrument used to scrap off tissue – may remove a lesion or take scrapings for examination Tissue curettes; not structured as the "shave" or biopsy and may leave some of the lesion behind severely disrupts the structure *see also* **Biopsy – shave technique**

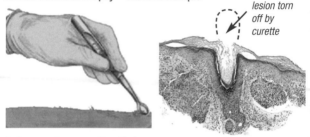

lesion torn off by curette

Cutaneous horn *see* **Keratin horn**

Cuticle keratinized part of the eponychium (skinfold at the base of the nail) also the outer covering of the HS *see also* **NAILS Nail anatomy**

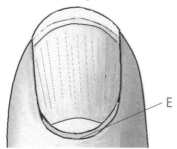

cutis- skin   D + E **adj cutaneous** *see also* **Subcutaneous**

Cyst nodule/tumor filled with liquid semi-solid material lined by epithelium – as opposed to unlined fluid in the pseudocyst

cyst- (SIST) bladder / fluid filled sac **adj cystic**

Cysts

> **Epithelial Cysts AKA Epidermoid cysts AKA Sebaceous cysts** *see* listed as Epitheloid cysts
>
> **Pilar Cysts AKA Tricholemmal cysts** Cyst formation as above but around a Scalp hair follicule present as a lump(s) when a person is combing their hair. These do not grow & are self limiting. Note the skin on the scalp is very tight which is why the growth is limited.

-cytes (SITES) mature cell types

cyto- (SĬ-toh) cellular

Cytokine any substance – generally small proteins made by a cell that affects the behaviour of other cells. Substance made by lymphocytes, act via specific cytokine receptors on the cells that they affect *see also* **Lymphokines, Interleukins (IL).**

Cytotoxic poisonous to cells – may cause cell death

Dactylitis AKA Sausage digit *Gk dactylos = finger*– If of the entire digit as seen in **Psoriasis**

Dandruff *see* **Dermatitis, Seborrheic dermatitis AKA Cradle cap** – dandruff of babies

Darier's disease *see* **Keratosis Follicularis**

Decubitus Ulcers Lt lying down AKA Bed sores AKA Pressure sore necrotic ulcer on areas under constant P - partic in paralysed &/or bedridden patients - involving skin & underlying subcut fat *see* **Ulcers.**

Deep plane refers to the deep dermal area - lower half with increased fat & decreased collagen fibres - collagen septa connect the skin with the underlying muscle in this area. *See also* **Hypodermis**

Demodicosis AKA Red Mange pimples/pustules at the hair exit (ie pores) on congested red skin due to over sensitivity or over population of **demodex folliculum** - SS hair loss, itchy H, rosacea-like appearance, crusted ELs.

Dendritic (stromal) cells AKA Langerhans cells AKA Antigen presenting cells BM-derived star-shaped/treelike tissue resident phagocytic cells – potent T cell stimulators using Ags attached to stimulate activity. Act in the skin as first line of defense.

dendro- tree-like formation

Dens *adj dentate* a tooth hence dentine & dental relating to teeth, denticulate having tooth-like projections *see also* **Odontoid**

Depilation removal of hair, generally referring to body hair

Depression a concavity on a surface

-derma relating to skin

Dercum's disease = Adiposis Dolorosa

Dermatitis in pathology / dermatopathology - any inflammatory condition of the skin (used in all pathological descriptions)

in dermatology - If of the skin *see also* **Eczema** (a term which is often used interchangeably by dermatologists) presents as red, scaly, puritic, ill-defined lesions which may be distributed to reflect the irritant substance & its contact with the skin **(Contact Dermatitis)** or may be associated with Atopy and hence is widespread,
Aetiology familial and associated with other IR diseases e.g. in the GIT or RT, asthma (Atopic dermatitis) –

Histo dermatitis can have diffuse or nodular patterns of inflammatory cells, which may be deep or superficial & may show more inflammation around the BVs of the area (perivascular) in the dermis, as the examples below show.

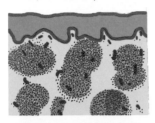
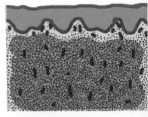

nodular pattern vs diffuse pattern

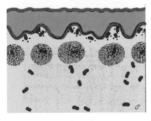
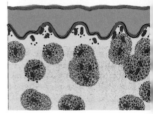

perivascular patterns of If superficial vs deep

contact dermatitis – localized red, inflamed skin

allergic contact dermatitis due to contact with an antigenic substance –which is unique to an individual

irritant contact dermatitis = eczema

due to contact with an irritant chemical direct injury e.g. bleach, formaldehyde , sprays – may be work related & localized e.g. face feet hands, precisely where there has been contact

Dermatitis Herpetiformis, AKA Duhring's Disease presents as very itchy bumps, pus bumps or tiny water blisters on the skin. The commonest areas are the elbows, knees, back of neck, upper back & near the base of the spine. It is associated with gluten intolerance – **Coeliac disease.**

Dermatitis Artifacta presents as bizarre shaped excoriations found in areas a person can reach and following no particular pattern of distribution – self inflicted sores scratched by the patient

Infected dermatitis when dermatitis is present it may become 2º infected with a *Staph Aureus* and develop a yellow weeping crust DD **Impetago**

Nappy rash AKA Diaper Dermatitis a form of **irritant dermatitis**

Nummular dermatitis lesions are round or coin shaped that turn red and itch. Aetiology unknown.

Phytophoto dermatitis a contact dermatitis from certain plants (psoralens)

Seborrhoeic dermatitis AKA Dandruff AKA Pityriasis Capitis redness & scaling on the hairy areas of the skin with loose white flakes – also **Cradle cap** when this is seen in infants

Aetiology normal skin yeast, **Pitysporium ovale**, which overgrows and loosens the skin

Stasis dermatitis presents as a swollen scaly greasy weeping skin eruption below the knee. The skin may be painful discolored red & inflamed. It can last for months or years. In long standing cases the skin may become very thick, immobile & fibrotic

Poor circulation in the legs, with reduced venous return causes fluid to build up & then to become inflamed

Complications include:

> 2º bacterial skin Ins
> Permanent scar formation & thickening, fibrotic changes **dermatoliposclerosis**.
> Chronic leg ulcers – Stasis ulcers
> In of underlying bone

Dermato-autoplasty skin grafts from the same person - different site

Dermatofibroma a common, firm, button-like growth, darker than the surrounding skin on the arms or legs, ± tender.

Aetiology an over-reactive scar from an insect bite see also **Keloid**

Dermatology the study of the skin

Dermatoliposclerosis *see* **Dermatitis, Stasis dermatitis**

Dermatomyositis presents as a mauve or pink skin rash on the face &/or neck & fingers with nail capillary dilatation associated with proximal muscle weakness

Dermatopathology the study of the diseases of the skin

Dermatoscope hand held magnifier (X10) with polarized light to closely examine skin lesions

Dermatosis any skin disease particularly non-inflammatory e.g. **Ashy dermatosis** – erythematous lesions with central grey macules which enlarge coalesce and leave grey marks on the skin

Dermis deep layer of the skin under the epidermis and its BM, composed of fibrocytes, BVs, Ns, and resident tissue immune cells - **2 sections upper papillary + lower reticular**

Dermo/ dermato-epithelial junction AKA Dermo-papillary junction junction b/n the upper epithelial layer & deeper CT dermal layer

Dermographism AKA dermatographism urticaria resulting from mild pressure on the skin – skin writing

Dermoid resembling skin

Desmocyte = fibrocyte supports and synthesizes collagen fibres in CT.

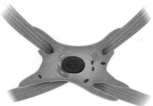

Desmosomes discrete area of cm for tight connections b/n cells, common in epithelial cells. Allows for cell to cell communication, cell adherence to the BM (an hemidesmosome) – important for the integrity of the skin, & other epithelial structures. Membranes are brought together via a series of filaments & adhering proteins *see also* **SKIN - epidermis**

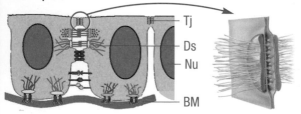

- Tj
- Ds
- Nu
- BM

Desquamation the sloughing off of cells from the SCorneum layer of the skin *see also* **Exfoliation**

Digital mucous cysts are cysts that grow near the end of the finger b/n the nail & 1st joint. They appear rubbery & translucent, containing jelly-like substance. ♀ > ♂

© A. L. Neill

Differentiation the changing of cells to become increasing specialized

Disc *adj discoid* (DISK-oyd) description of skin lesion - disc-like *see also* **Nummular**

Discoid Lupus Erythematosus (DLE) presents as red, scaly lesions on the sun exposed areas of the body (face, back of hands, arms & upper chest). Unlike SLE no systemic disease is involved, but the crusts when removed may leave changed pigmentation in the skin & scarring. Aetiology AI disease of the skin.

Distal further away from the axial skeleton (opposite of Proximal)

Dolor pain 1 of the 5 cardinal signs of IF

dorsi-back

dys- (DIS) *Gk bad sign* abnormal, bad, difficult, disorganized, painful (opposite to eu)

Dysplasia (DIS-play-zee-yah) abnormal growth of tissues or cells

Dysplastic naevus AKA Clark's nevus AKA Abnormal Mole. presents as tan, brown, or dark brown mole with indistinct borders.

Aetiology familial, and may be precancerous. *See also* **Naevus**

Duhring's Disease *see* **Dermatitis Herpetiformis**

Dyshidrosis *see* **Pompholyx**

Dyskeratosis premature keratinization of the cells

Ecchymosis (ek-EE-moh-sis) small haemorrhagic round bluey purple spot on the skin or MM *see* **Bruise, Haemotoma, Petechia**

Eccrine (EK-reen) gland specific type of exocrine gland which secretes by pinocytosis not damaging the secreting cell, re skin -generally referring to sweat glands, consists of coiled regions where the secretion is produced and straight connecting tube to the surface, where the secretion is concentrated – much like the renal tubules - depending upon the fluid balance of the body, note the changes in the epithelial lining – coiled base cells change from columnar to cuboidal cells – straight tubular cells - cuboidal *see also* **Apocrine, Holocrine, MT SKIN – Skin appendages**

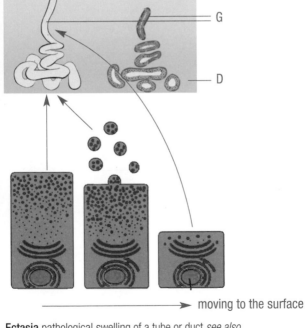

E

BM

Du

G

D

→ moving to the surface

Ectasia pathological swelling of a tube or duct *see also* *telangectasia*

Ectyma Grangrenosum (IK-tï-muh) painful tender ulceration which progresses from haemorrhagic vesicles to necrotic ulcers

Eczema (EX-smu) *Gk ekzein – to bubble out* AKA Dermatitis *both terms are used interchangeably* and it is by common usage that one is used more than another – but the term DERMATITIS is used more in legal settings. It is the preferred term and the correct dermatopathological term. –

presents as a red vesicular rash which is itchy. It recurs and is longstanding – it does not scale, become brighter on scratching and may not be symmetrical although it can be widespread. DD **Psoriasis**

Discoid Eczema = Nummular dermatitis presents as well-defined crusty blistering plaques with a red scaly base on the legs hands or body

Dyshidrotic Eczema = Pompholyx

Distribution of Eczema / Dermatitis in adults and children
Flexural surfaces, hands & feet are common to both groups, but the head moves to the neck and genital areas in adults. 80% of children with eczema develop asthma ± allergies

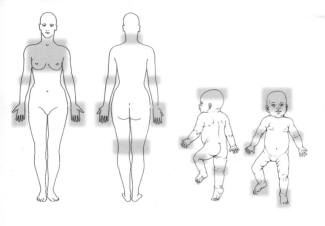

Edema AS Oedema

Effector cells describes those lymphocytes which develop from naïve lymphocytes after initial activation by Ag. They mediate the removal of pathogens from the body w/o further differentiation. Naïve lymphocytes & memory lymphocytes must differentiate &/or proliferate before they become effector lymphocytes.

Effluvium a shedding of hair –

>**anogen effluvian** shed hair due to chemotherapy; actively growing hair is lost

>**telogen effluvian** shed hair due to shock either physiological e.g. diet/hormonal or emotional; resting hair is lost cycle is accelerated into catagen

Elephantiasis *see* Filiaris

Endogenous growing from w/n tissues or cells

Ephelis (e-FELL-is) *pl ephelides* (e-FELL-ee-dees) **AKA freckle**, flat brown circular macule on the skin

Epidermal Naevus *see* Naevus

Epithelial cells – cells from the germinal layer of the ectoderm – used to describe lining cells – always resting on a basement membrane (BM) & skin cells *see also* **Keratinocytes**

All epithelial skin cells rest on a BM, and form a progressive layer where they are connected and communicate with each other.

Most epithelial cells have occlusive zones (OZ) to prevent passage of any materials, adherent zones (AZ) to keep them in line and together. AZs are made up of individual Desmosomes which are also found all over the cell as spot connections (Ds) joining the cell membranes (CM) together & the cell to the BM connected via actin filaments (A).

Gap junctions (GJ) are present to facilitate intercellular communications.

Without these connections epithelial cells will migrate as a line until they can be restored – they do not function as individual cells. This is important in wound healing processes.

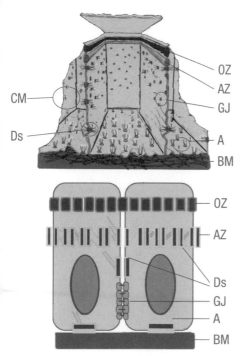

Labels: OZ, AZ, GJ, CM, A, Ds, BM

Simple epithelium is single layered

simple columnar – lining the GIT with moistening Goblet cells (Gc) which discharge mucous & keep the layer moist

simple cuboidal – lining the eccrine glands of the skin & other exocrine glands

simple squamous – lining BVs & lymphatics

see also MT SKIN - epidermis and cell types

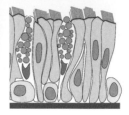

some epithelial cells appear multilayered but are not. Every cell actually lies on the BM even though it appears no to do so e.g. as in the **Pseudostratified columnar epithelium** of the RT

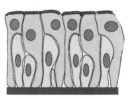

some epithelial cells are highly flexible changing their shapes to the demands of their site as in the **Transitional epithelial** lining of the bladder

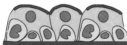

empty bladder ➔ *full bladder*

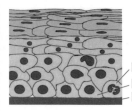

Stratified epithelium is multilayered & the epithelium leaves the BM to move upwards and slough off. However only the basal cells (Bc) attached to the BM undergo mitosis (Mc).

Mc
Bc
BM

Stratified squamous cells may contain little or no keratin in the upper layers, with the nuclei persisting throughout as in these cells of the oesophagus & other MMs. These are moist sites and do not need to act as a waterproof barrier. This pattern of cells on the skin is pathological – *see* **Parakeratosis**

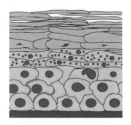

Normal skin is a **stratified squamous epithelium** – with dead cell skeletons in the upper layers heavily invested with keratin (SCorneum), but with tight connections in the lower live layers to act as a barrier b/n the inside & the outside

Epithelial Cysts AKA Sebacious cysts develop from a comedo with sebaceous gland involvement, present as smooth surfaced yellow-white nodules just under the skin with or w/o a black punctum or pore.

Incidence - common in young males – in neck and beard area, if the cysts are removed – they tend to return.

Aetiology - Sebaceous glands grow until so large the centre becomes necrotic, sebum is trapped from escaping & a tender lump develops, grows & becomes painful. **DD Lipoma**

Deeper Epithelial cysts are usually skin colour on the surface. They present as a lump on the torso (but may be anywhere) in the young adult. Shed skin cells are trapped in the cyst cavity & continue to grow & build up into a cavity formation, rather than to shed. similar to a large Blackhead – They are common & familial increasing in number & size with time, & may become infected. They tend to reform when removed & can become painful. *see also* **MT SKIN – epidermal appendages**

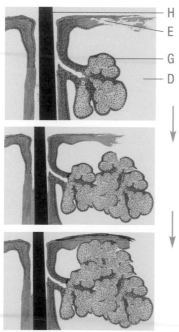

H
E
G
D

Epithelioid epithelial like cells or T which have changed to look more like the epithelium- as in epitheloid histiocyte of the **granuloma**

Epithelium (epi-THEE-lee-um) – collective term for layers of keratinocytes on the skin

Eponychium (epon-NIK-ee-um) fold of normal epidermis at the nail bed

Epulis (ep-OO-lis) **AKA Gumboil** congenital tumour of the gums particularly of the Maxilla

Erosion an area of partial loss of the epithelium on the skin or mucous membrane, often due to deterioration of a blister

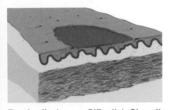

Erysipalis (er-ee-SIP-alis) *Gk pella = skin eryth = red* acute supf cellulitis involving dermal lymphocytes due to bacterial In

    erysipeloid an AIf reaction to a bacterial In from a puncture wound which then swells the affected digit and causes an elevated ring border – gyrate border with vesicles and may compromise the BS of the appendage if it includes the whole circumference

Erythema (er-EE-them-ah) *adj. erythematous, Gk erythema – flush upon the skin* redness – noun, eruption of skin with dilated dermal BVs & oedema – one of the 5 cardinal signs of If – blanchable redness = pressure on the skin will cause the redness to diminish, as opposed to **purpura**.

It is also used to describe a number of skin changes with redness as a major feature of the presentation. It is present in any If of the skin.

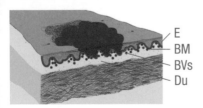

    E
    BM
    BVs
    Du

Erythema Infectiosum AKA Fifth Disease AKA Slapped Cheek disease presents as a red rash on the face that gives a slapped cheek appearance, which extends in 2-3 days to a fish net like pattern of redness on the arms & trunk, due to a viral In. Mild and self resolving it is only important in pregnant women where the foetus may be compromised. It is highly contagious

Erythema multiforme (EM) a characteristic pattern of target or Iris lesions characterise this - the lesion has a central vesicular core on an erythematosus plaque, these appear all over the body not sparing the heels palms or mouth. There are mild & severe forms.

EM Major = Steven Johnson syndrome = toxic epidermal necrolysis has severe involvement of the MM with skin sloughing and 2° In common.

EM minor is commoner and is a similar but less severe form , and has various aetiologies – idiopathic – unknown – over reaction to Ins and viruses and an hypersensitive reaction of the BVs to the Herpes Simplex virus.

Erythematosis redness due to BV engorgement rather than an If process.
 see **Discoid Lupus Erythematosis (DLE)**
 see **Systemic Lupus Erythematosis (SLE)**

Eruptive Xanthoma presents as multiple yellow to red bumps which appear in "showers" on the skin. caused by tiny accumulations of fat droplets in resident cells of the skin. This type of eruption has been associated with underlying medical conditions such as: DM & disorders of the blood fats.

If an underlying cause is found, treatment of the underlying disease may result in clearing of the xanthomas. *See also* **Xanthoma**

Erythrasma bacterial In of the flexural surfaces – generally involving them all, presenting as a brown-orange scaley plaque – similar to **Tinea Cruris**

Erythroderma *adj erythrodermic* abnormal redness of the skin

Erythroplasia AKA erythroplakia red papules on MMs.

Erythroplasia of Queyrat AKA Bowen's disease epithelial dysplasia – small red circumscribed red plaques regarded as CIN – cells pleomorphic found on the glans penis or vulva *see also* **Keratoacanthoma.**

Eschar *Gk eschara – scab adj escharotic* a piece of dead tissue sloughed off from injury partic burns, gangrenous processes & fungal Ins – e.g. Black Eschar may cause the circulation to be compromised and should always be treated seriously

Exclamation point hairs = ! hair pathenomonic sign of alopecia areata – short hairs on the edge of bald areas that have thin exiting shafts *see also* **Alopecia, MT HAIR – Hair loss**

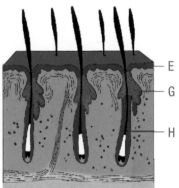

- E
- G
- H

Exoriation a scratch mark which has scored the epidermis ± penetrated beyond the BM e.g. mild trauma, as in picking of sores, nail diggin

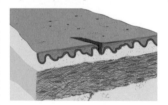

Exfoliation AKA desquamation removal of the surface corneocytes. This occurs naturally controlled by proteolytic degradation of Ds but is accelerated by chemical peels and dermabrasion, to encourage a foster turnover of epithelial cells

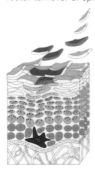

Exogen short phase where hair falls out *see also* **Hair cycle**

External Auditory Meatus (EAM) ear hole

Extracellular (ec) outside the cell

Extrafibrillar matrix *see* **Ground substance**

Fabry's disease = Angiokeratoma corporis diffusum

Factitious (FAK-tish-us) artificial, unnatural, not naturally occurring – as in an atopic rash due to application of a stimulant

Fascia (FASH-ee-ah) *Lt = a band* a sheet or band of fibrous T deep in the skin covering & attaching to deeper tissues

Fascicle (FAS-ih-kul) small bundle

Fc receptor the section of the cm which binds the Fc portion of the Ab (IL).

Felting matting threads – hairs which are dry and with irregular structures may felt – *see* **kinky hair**

Fever a generalized ⬆ in body temperature due to an ⬆ BF, which may be due to the body's IfR

Fibrino-inflammatory exudates due to IfR with both fibrin & inflammatory components

Fibrous papule of the nose *see* **Papule**

Fibroblast (Fb) an immature progenitor cell found in all CT, capable of mitosis, migration, movement. They develop into fibrocytes **(Fc)**.

Fibrocyte mature fibre producing cell = mature fibroblast – spindle shaped cell producing either collagen **(Co)** or elastin **(e)** fibres via secretion of monomer units **(m)** which assemble outside the cell into long fibres, which are then maintained by the fibrocytes. Note with age the number of fibrocytes & hence the fibres hence compromising the integrity & strength of the dermis, and making the skin frailer and more vulnerable to tearing – *see also* **MT SKIN – Skin aging overview, Dermis**

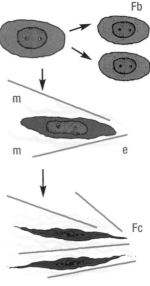

Fibro-epithelial polyps *see* **Acrocordon**

Fibromatosis formation of a fibrous tumour-like nodule or multiple nodules from the deep fascia – or subcutaneous tissue

Fibrosis (FĪ-broh-sis) increased fibrous T – collagen fibres – this can occur in all organs – often replacing normal T

With skin this occurs in the dermis – and may be disorganized collagen post Alf or generalized thickening as a reaction to Clf. Fibrous tissue constantly turns over and becomes more organized and less cellular over time. Extreme localized fibrosis becomes scar / keloid material. *see also* **Keloid, Scar**

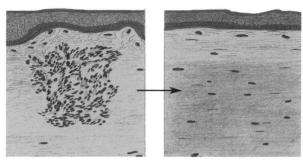

Fibroxanthoma (FY- broh-zanth-mu) deposition of fat in the dermal macrophages associated with fibrous over-growth DD **BCC**

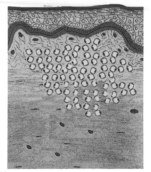

Fifth Disease *see* **Erythema Infectiosum** – one of the original "six diseases of erythematous rashes"

Filaggrin a protein which binds to keratin fibres in the skin and acts to maintain an impermeable skin water barrie *see* **lamellae bodies MT SKIN - structure water barrier**

Filiariasis AKA Philiariasis (FIL-ee-ar-eye-a-sis) – a parasitic disease where the infective agent , nemotodes – roundworms, transmitted by mosquitoes lodge in lymphatics and then block them with their fibrous growths causing swelling of the skin & subcutaneous tissues of the legs to such an extent it is also called elephantiasis. Other dependant areas may also be infected and swell dramatically eg the scrota

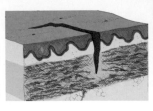

Filiform thread-shaped

Fissure (FISH-er) a narrow slit or gap from cleft - in skin a split through to the dermis

Fitzpatrick skin type the commonest scheme used to classify a person's skin type by their response to sun exposure – *see also* **MT SKIN – Skin photo-types**

Flushing *see* **Blushing**

Follicle *adj follicular pl folliculi* **Lt** *folliculus = little leather bag (from follis = leather bag)* very small excretory duct or gland e.g. folliculus pila = hair follicle

Folliculitis If of the hair follicles presents as an eruption of skin that surrounds a hair or hair pore. Many red bumps or "pus" bumps are seen. Frequently a hair is seen coming out of the center of an individual bump. Any part of the skin can be involved except for the palms & soles, but commonly: the LL, UL, axilla & pubic area are involved *see also* **pseudofolliculitis**

    folliculitis barbae – folliculitis which involves the beard/facial area on a male

Folium (FOH-lee-um) *pl folia adj foliacious* **Lt** *folium = leaf* description of any leaf like structure as in keratin leaf like over hanging in disrupted bullae

Freckle = Ephelis (>5mm) – flat brown mark level with the skin < 3mm *see also* **Macule** (>5mm)

Fox-Fordyce disease *see* **Apocrine**

Furuncle AKA Boil painful, red, pus-filled lump in the skin from an In in an HF. If a punctum develops then the pus can drain relieving the discomfort, but often due to the IfR the amount of necrotic T results in a scar on healing. ***Staph Aureus*** is the commonest infective agent.

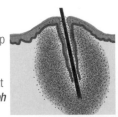

Gamma Gk letter shaped like a "Y" and used to describe shapes of Igs.

Gene (JEEN) a functional unit of heredity that occupies a specific place on a chromosome. and directs the formation of a protein.

Gene expression the detectable effect of a gene.

Genital Herpes *see* **Herpes Progenitalis**

Genodermatoses genetically determined skin disorder 3 distinct types: single gene inheritance, polygenic & chromosomal e.g. epidermal naevi all those skin diseases which have a familial component

German measles *see* **Rubella**

Gingiva (JIN-jiv-uh) *Lt gum* gums

Glabella *Lt glabellus – smooth adj glabrous* that region b/n the nose & eyebrows generally used to indicate hairlessness as in glabrous skin of the lips, palms & soles

Glomerulus *Lt – little knot* knot generally referring to BVs which have one incoming vessel – then branch into many and return to have one exiting vessel as in the kidney glomeruli

Glomus *Lt knot* knot

Glomus bodies arterio-venous aa of BVs found in palms / soles / tips of digits / nail-beds responsible for temp control in these regions (G)

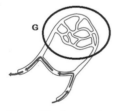

Glossa *Gk glossa = tongue see also* **Lingua**

Graft tissue or organ implantation or transplantation – ***skin graft*** for transplanatation of skin from one place or person to another

Granulocytes cells with granules
2 types in the BS / Immune system - WBCs with granules
    see **Neutrophils, WBCs**
    in the skin – epithelial cells accumulating keratin granules –
    SGranulosum – granulocytes *see* **Keratinocytes**

Granuloma (Gran-YOU- low- mah) a smooth jelly orange-yellow papule nodule which microscopically appears as an aggregation of MNCs; a collection of modified macrophages – epitheloid cells, histiocytes surrounded by lymphocytes ± giant cells and fibrocytes – attempting to wall off the area from the surrounding tissue, a granuloma is a feature of Clf *see also* **Granulomatosis**

Granulomatosis – the process of forming granulomae a response in Clf when there is no resolution of the process.

In the skin this process may develop in a number of different cellular patterns depending upon the causative agents – and in some cases these patterns are interchangeable.

A = sarcoidal granuloma when there are only epithelioid histiocytes (EH) & Giant cells (GC) present - in response to inert foreign bodies (FB).

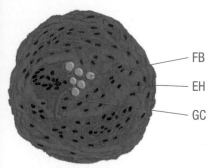

— FB
— EH
— GC

A¹= palisading granuloma - when the epithelioid histiocytes (EH) are arranged in a fence-like manner – later form of A as occurs in rheumatoid nodules

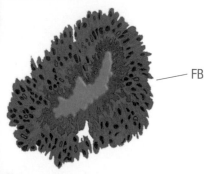

— FB

A² = interstitial granuloma – when there are collagen fibres (Co) dispersed around and through the Histiocytes – a variant of A when there is a fibrotic response

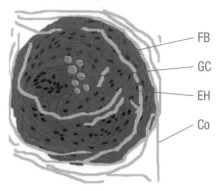

— FB

— GC

— EH

— Co

B = tuberculoid granuloma when there is a dense lymphocytic (L) mantle of cells around the centre – in response to bacterial infective agents and necrotic tissue (N)

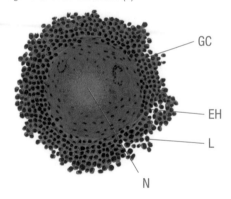

— GC

— EH

— L

N

C = suppuratives granuloma - when there is an abscess process concurrently occurring and there are a number of PMNs & necrotic material also present generally in the centre - in response to fungal Ins

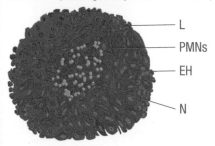

- L
- PMNs
- EH
- N

Granuloma Annulare presents as individual discs / rings of inflamed T on the dorsal extremities of children which expand, developing a pale centre and then resolve over weeks to months

Aetiology: insect bite, trauma or idiopathic which has an Immune overreaction in hypersensitive individuals **DD fungal skin In e.g. Ringworm, Nummular Dermatitis, Tinea, Lichen Planus, Sarcoid nodules.**

Granulosis the extent of the SGranulsum layer in the skin – normal number of granulocytes

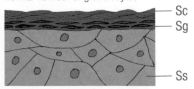

- Sc
- Sg
- Ss

hypergranulosis – increased number of granulocytes

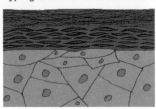

hypogranulosis – decreased number of granulocytes – may be associated with a defective SCorneum

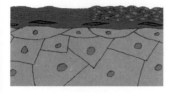

Groove long pit or furrow

Ground substance AKA Extrafibrillar matrix – refers to the material in T which is not fibrous or cellular – seen in the Dermis and other T. particuarly cartilage.

Growth factors natural substances produced by the body or obtained from food that promote growth and development by directing cell maturation and differentiation and by mediating maintenance and repair of tissues

Gumma chronic focal area of If due to tertiary syphilis – resembles a granuloma = syphiloma

Guttate drop-like used to describe types of psoriatic lesion distribution

Guttate Psoriasis *see* **Psoriasis**

Gyrus *pl gyri Lt gyros = round*, circle, curved

haemo (HEEM-oh) AS hemo- referring to blood

Haemochromotosis – a disease of excessive iron storage in the body – manifests on the skin as a deep pigmentation often the person appears "bronzed" because oxidized iron is deposited in the skin.

Haematoma (HEEM-u-toh-mah) *Gk haeme = blood:-oma = tumor/lump* Bruise, Black heel, Blood blister localized coloured lump of extravasated B in the skin due to trauma – spontaneously heals changing colours to relate haemoglobin breakdown red, purple, blue, green, yellow

Hailey–Hailey disease *see* **benign familial chronic pemphigous**

Hair *Gk- thrix / Lt- pilus hair on the skin = pilus /* hair on the scalp capilli – hair cycle 3 stages

types Terminal - this is the thicker coarser hair found on the head buried deep in the subcutaneous fat (Su) with a strong BS

Vellus - this is the finer lighter hair found on most parts of the body attached to pilus erectus muscle (Mu)

Androgenic - this is the Vellus hair which develops under the influence of androgens to take on some of the characteristics of Terminal hair in specific areas e.g. the axilla, face, pubic region, & to a lesser extent – the arms, back, chest, legs,

within these main types are several subgroups – *see* **HAIR – Hair types**

terminal hair   vellus hair

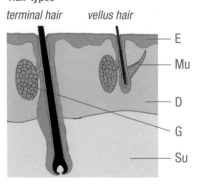

Club hair = hair root surrounded by bullous enlargement prior to shedding

Exclamation point hair = bulbo-atrophy ± attenuation – sign of alopecia areata – *see also* **Exclamation hair**

Ingrown hair = burrowing hair – growing under the skin not able to emerge causing irritation, may develop after plucking – epithelium grows over while the new hair is developing – maybe development of folliculitis (this may occur with vellus hair)

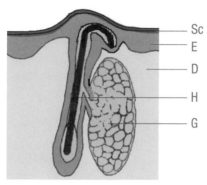

Sc
E
D
H
G

Halo Naevus *see* **Naevus**

Hamartoma any congenital defect of tissue or organ

Hangnail AKA Agnail *Eng from – anguished nail* piece of skin torn from the cuticle or surrounding skin of the nail

Aetiology dry cracked skin *see also* **Paronychia Whitlow**

Herpangina an acute

Head Lice AKA Nits *see* **Pediculosis Capitis**

Hemidesmosome *see* **Desmosome**

hemo- AS haemo

Henoch – Scholein purpura *see* **Purpura**

Herald Patch *see* **Pityriasis Rosea**

Herpangina an acute infectious disease with vesico-ulcerative lesions on the MMs = **vesicular pharyngitis**

Herpes *Gk herpein – to creep* name of Herpes viridae group of DNA viruses which cause latent and recurring Ins in specific sites. The virus can lie dormant for years often in the local NR undetected but still shedding virions & so still contagious & then reappear as a severe florid lytic presentation, presenting with acutely painful vesicles in the affected site.

There are 8 viruses in this family which infect humans and they are site specific. Sites of In include: the eye, skin, mouth etc

Herpes Progenitalis AKA Genital herpes (Herpes is also often used to refer to this In) viral skin In of the genital region.

Herpes Simplex type 3 AKA Herpes Zoster - Shingles (adults) AKA Chicken Pox (Children)

Herpetiform – like Herpes but w/o the virus

hidro- *Gk hidros = sweat* relating to sweat

Hidrocystoma benign tumour of the sweat glands appears as a translucent painless swelling **DD Blister**

Hidrosis AS Hydrosis = hyperhidrosis excessive sweating in the eccrine sweat glands

Hirsute (HER-suit) *Gk hirsutus = shaggy* hairy

Hirsiutism having abundant, excessive hair referring to a female with hair >2cm on arms, upper back, chest, chin, lips ± male body hair pattern seen on a female, ± ⬆ androgen levels *see also* **Trichosis Polytrichosis**

Histamine vasoactive amine stored in mast-cell granules – basophilic histiocytes

histio-/hist-/histeo *Gk histos = web tissues*

Histiocyte (hist-EE-oh-site) *Gk histio- tissue = phagocytic tissue cell* a cell in the tissues which is immunologically active, derived from the BM and phagocytic. In Clf they may undergo epithelioid transformation *see also* **Granulomatosis**

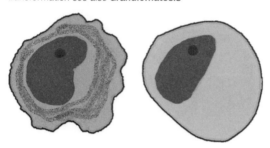

Hive fluid filled epidermis *see also* **Wheal, Urticaria**

Holocrine glands a secretory gland where the product is formed inside the cytoplasm; secretion causes the disruption of the cell membrane and destruction of the cell e.g. Sebaceous glands *see also* **Apocrine, Eccrine & Mercrine.**

Hordeolum (hord-EE-oh-lum) *Lt barely grain AKA Stye* small pustule on the eyelid – folliculitis of the eyelash hair

Hormone *Gk hormaein = to spur on* a substance secreted n the body having a regulatory affect on organs & tissues

Horn AKA Cutaneous horn AKA Keratin horn benign localized outgrowth of keratin from SCorneum - incidence ⬆ with age & sun exposure

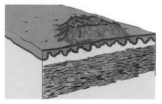

Humectants AKA Desiccants = hygroscopic molecules which attract water from the atmosphere e.g. urea, sodium lactate naturally occurring body substances secreted onto the skin & glycerin – used in skin care, properties include : ⬇ transepidermal water loss, ⬆ production of ceramide, ⬆ skin plasticity

Hutchinson's freckle see **Leartigo maligna melanoma**

hyper- (HIGH –per) over the top / above

Hyperhidrosis excessive sweating in the axilla groin palms &/or soles *see also* **Hidrosis**

Hyperkeratosis horny skin; an overgrowth of the SCorneum *see also* **Bunion, Callus, Keratoma, Keratosis**

Hypertrichosis excessive hair growth *see also* **Polytrichia, Trichosis**

hypo- underneath / below

Hypodermis AKA Subcutaneous Tissue AKA Subcutis AKA Deep Dermis this term indicates the dermis layer below the dense collagen fibres of the upper dermis and is generally filled with fat cells and collagen septae

It can be confusing as these terms are used by many in different ways – image below clarifies the situation

Hyponychium AKA Quick thickened epidermis which goes from the floor of the nailfold to the undersurface of the nail *see also* **Subungual**

Ichthyosis (IK-thee-oh-sis) - *Gk fish* generalized term for any aberrant keratinization – generally dry scaly skin

Aetiology congenital – *crocodile skin / fish skin*

Ideopathic of unknown origin

Immune (IM-youn) *Lt – immunis = to free, to exempt* free from the possibility of acquiring a certain disease or infection

Immune Complexes Ab/Ag combinations used to stimulate the IR

Immune response (IR) any response made by an organism to defend itself against pathogens.

Immune system a coordinated system of cells, tissues, & soluble products that constitutes the body's defense against invasion by non-self entities, e.g. infectious and inert agents & tumour cells.

Immunity a state of biological defense using an entire system of cells, structures & substances - immune system - to combat infectious agents or biological invasion, in either a non-specific (innate immunity) or specific way (adaptive immunity).

Immunoglobulins (Ig) = antibodies Ab proteins involved in the IR either secreted or fixed on the cell surface

Immunology the study of the cell, tissues, organs & substances involved in the body's defense against attack by microbes, foreign bodies or tumours, & any adverse consequences of the IR *see also* **Inflammation**.

Impetigo (IM-pet-ar-goh) contagious pyoderma due to *Grp A Streptococcus* or *Staph Aureus Ins*

Inclusion any foreign or heterogeneous substance w/n a cell not introduced as a result of trauma.

Induration *Lt induartio - to harden* long standing dermal thickening (fibrous induration) and hardening produced by excessive dermal collagen – or other infiltrate

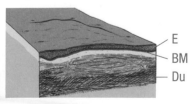

E
BM
Du

Inferior under

Inflammation = Inflammatory Response (IfR) the body's stereotypical response to damage indicated by 5 cardinal signs: dolor = pain; calor = heat; tumor = swelling; rubor = redness; function laesa = loss of function

> **acute** immediate, severe, short lived, predominant cells PMNs
> **chronic** slow onset, long lasting, associated with long term irritation & healing, predominant cell types MNCs

Inter between

Interleukins (inter-LOO-kins) (IL) "communication b/n leucocytes" *see also* Lymphokines often designated IL-X with X a number indicating specific characteristics of the signals instigated by this IL

Intertrigo *Gk terere = to rub* superficial odiferous discolouring dermatitis due to opposing skin surfaces – as in the axilla under the breast or groin with obesity being a predisposing factor

Intra within

Intracellular inside the cell

Introitus an orifice or point of entry to a cavity or space.

Itching is a symptom, skin is irritated but not painful – may be caused by low grade T hypoxia & associated with:

> dermatitis
> drug reaction
> dry skin
> hives
> insect bites
> ring worm
> Ins bacterial / fungal /viral

see also **Puritis**

-itis inflammation of

Keloid (KEE- loyd) *Gk Kelis = blemish* sharply elevated progressively enlarging scar due to the formation of excessive collagen in the healing process extends beyond the original scar area *see also* **scar**

Aetiology – unknown, familial, ethnic, post-trauma, post surgery – commoner in darker races

commonest sites – back, chest, ear, jawline, shin, note areas where the skin is drawn tightly over the bone

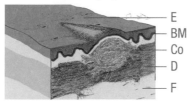

E
BM
Co
D
F

kerat- / kerato- (KER-at-oh) *Gk keratos = horn horny AKA cerat- /cerato-*

Keratin a family of fibrous structural proteins, which are the key structural material making up the outer layer of human skin & the major protein of Hair & Nails. Produced as monomers they assemble into bundles to form intermediate filaments and then tough unmineralized tissue (note this is the covering of some tablets – as keratin is not digested by gastric juices but can be dissolved by duodenal peptidases)

Keratin horn *see* **Horn**

Keratinocyte epithelial cell which accumulates keratin granules in their cytoplasm - predominant cell type of the epidermis, note the keratinocytes has a number of shapes described in terms of epithelial cell structure in diagram showing the progression of the keratocytes to maturity & death *see also* **Corneocyte, Epithelial cells, Epithelium SKIN – Epidermis**

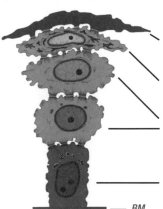

Sc = dead corneocytes full of keratin & b/n keratin strands

Sl = clear layer of dead keratinocytes with increasing keratin intracellularly

Sg = dying squamous epithelial cells filled with keratin granules granulocytes

Ss = shrinking spikey cells spinocytes (prickle cells) cuboidal to squamous with strong TJCs b/n the cells layer of waterproofing of the skin

Sb = cuboidal actively dividing epithelial cells sitting on the BM - which move upwards

BM

Keratoacanthoma AKA Bowen's disease a locally distorted expanding epithelium which resembles an SCC – is considered precancerous SCC presents on sun exposed areas as a thick growth that has a central crusted plug that may look like a horn. Pink/Red, it often has a central crater or horny plug. It can grow up to 20 cm = Giant keratoacanthoma. It may clear spontaneously, but this is less likely in those with multiple lesions *see also* **SCC**

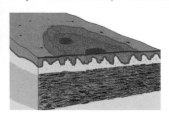

Keratoderma thickening of the soles of the feet mainly in females particularly the edge of the heel & ball of the feet –

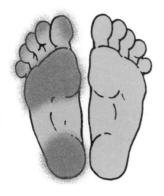

Keratolytic dissolving or lysis of the SCorneum layer of the skin resulting in softening of the horny layer – e.g. Salicylic acid creams

Keratolysis adj keratolytic (KER-at-oh-lit-ik) the dissolving or lysis of the SCorneum layer of the skin resulting in its softening

Pitted keratolysis non-bacterial odouriferous in of the soles of the feet.

Aetiology bacterial overgth due to closed in shoes & keratin dissolution

characeteristic feature : appearance of pits on the soles. assoc. with (hyperhydrosis) of the feet.

Keratosis AKA Hyperkeratosis hyperplasia of the SCorneum which causes horny outgrowths on the skin – e.g. **keratin horn, wart**

note histologically this occurs in defined patterns

the Orthokeratoses – where the SCorneum is thickened but essentially normal & Parakeratosis – where the nuclei are extended into the SCorneum

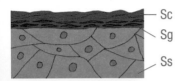

— Sc
— Sg
— Ss

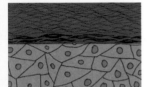

normal hyperkeratosis - basketweave pattern

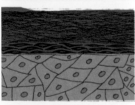

compact orthokeratosis - corneocytes are denser but normal pattern is maintained

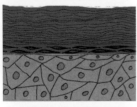

laminated orthokeratosis - compacted corneocytes as in the normal palms & soles

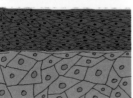

parakeratosis - no SLucidum no true SCorneum as the nuclei persist to the surface & all layers are thicker

Actinic keratoses (AK) AKA Solar Keratoses AKA Precancers AKA Sun damage spots AKA Senile keratoses red-brown, scaly patches, sensitive to touch & occurring on sun exposed areas: the face, scalp, ears, neck, hands & arms.

adults > 30yrs **DD Lentigo, SCC**

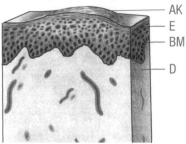

AK
E
BM
D

Keratosis Follicularis AKA Darier's disease consists of dark red greasy smelly skin patches on the scalp, hands, nails and feet. It is an autosomal dominant disease due to defective Ds keratin, which stops the epidermal cells from adhering to each other properly

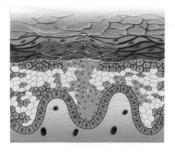

keratosis pilaris appears as multiple rough bumps on the back of the arms, & other body areas such as the cheeks and thighs; generally resolves with age >40 yrs.

seborrheaic keratoses overgrowth & protrusion of the SBasale with basal cells protruding through the skin and having a warty waxy texture look like they are stuck on the skin

stucco keratoses multiple keratotic papules found on the distal lower acral extremities of elderly adults ♂ > ♀. The lesions appear stuck on but due to friction may grow out in a spire from the skin and look like roof tiles. The SSpinosum and SGranulosum layers grow through the SCorneum and lie on the surface. The amount of keratin in the cells determines the greasiness.

uncommon

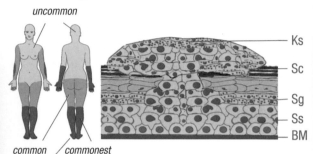

— Ks
— Sc
— Sg
— Ss
— BM

common / commonest
absent on soles of feet

Kerion is an inflamed, thickened, pus-filled area on the scalp or nape of the neck, and it is sometimes accompanied by a fever 2^0 to ringworm or In by any of the normal geophytes & as an overreaction to them *see also* **Ringworm**

Kimara's Disease = Angiolymphoid Hyperplasia fatal recessive X-linked disease of Copper metabolism - female carriers have wirey white fragile hair

Kinky Hair disease AKA Menke's syndrome fatal recessive X-linked disease of copper metabolism - female carrier always has wirey, white, fragile hair

-kines stimulation, activation &/or division of cells

Koebner phenomenon AKA Isomorphic response response of the skin to form linear lesions at sites of injury – which are not due to auto-inoculation or direct In as observed in warts – but are 2^0 to the scratching and not direct In as in **Psoriasis** – traumatic lines cause the psoriatic condition to flare up in those sites later.

Also occurs in **Lichen Planus, Vitiligo** and other AI diseases *see also* **Pathergy Psoriasis**

Koplik spots spots which look like grains of sand on a red base, pathoenogenic of measles

Labium *Lt lip pl labia adj Labial* lips / pertaining to the lips – used to describe lips, on the face, and the Labia majora & minora of the vagina *see also* **Vulva**

Lacrima *Lt tear adj Lacrimal* related to tears and tear drops.

Lamellar bodies (LB) AKA membrane coated granules AKA Keratinosomes wrt skin oblong tubulo-vesicular organelles synthesized by the GA and related to lysosomes. They appear in granular keratinocytes where they are exported extra cellularly and coat the surface corneocytes of Sc contributing to the skin-water-barrier. These bodies appear anywhere there needs to be a separation from the cell & its environment, eg in the GIT & RT

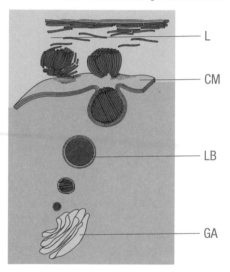

L

CM

LB

GA

Lamina *(pl. laminae)* a plate as in different plates of the skin *see also* **Stratum**

Langerhan's cells *see* **Dendritic cells of the skin** *see also* **MT SKIN – Epidermis cell types**

Lanugo (Lan–OO-goh) *Lt lana = wool down*, fine hair embryonic hair appearing in the 3rd month of gestation v fine hair with large papillae - present in severe states of malnutrition *see also* **HAIR - Types**

Laser treatments *see* **Selective Photothermolysis**

Lentigo (LEN–tee-goh) *pl Lentigines* **(LEN-tig–inees) AKA Liver Spots** present in adults as brown flat pigmented macule surrounded by normal skin *see also* **Macules**

Lentigo Maligna (melanoma) a flat, mottled, tan-to-brown freckle-like spots with irregular borders, on elderly people. Typically they enlarge slowly 5-15 years before becoming invasive *see also* **Melanoma**.

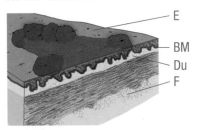

Lentigo Simplex AKA Simple Lentigo AKA Juvenile Lentigo present from birth as a single or multiple lesions – not influenced by sun exposure – may become more numerous or resolve spontaneously – do not become malignant

Senile Lentigo AKA Age Spots increase with age often show an heredity pattern

Solar Lentigo seen on sun exposed areas, face, back of hands, arms, chest and lower legs, but which do not darken after exposure to the sun unlike freckles. **DD Solar Keratosis, Freckles**

Lesion any single area of altered skin single or multiple *see also* **Rash**

leuco-/ leuko- AKA luco /luko (LOO- koh) white, pale, clear

Leucocyte = white blood cell (WBC)

Leucoplakia a persistent white hyperkeratotic plaque in the mouth (MM) due to epithelial dysplasia or CIN

Lice *see* **Pediculosis Capitis**

Lichen (Lï-ken) *Gk leichen = moss* thickened, pink- purple, itchy bumps on the skin & MMs of the ankles, elbows, genitalia, nails, tongue & wrists. White lines appearing in the bumps are called Wickham's striae

Rarely presents on the scalp – causing scars & irreversible hair loss

On the genitals lumps may be very red & painful

Aetiology hypersensitive reaction due to past lf, or foreign substances, ± familial, ± hepatitis C

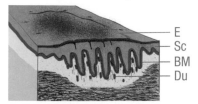

— E
— Sc
— BM
— Du

exaggeration of the epithelial markings & ⬆ papilla in the dermo-epithelial junction with induced vertical collagen fibre formation

Lichen Planus 3-5mm bumps on the skin as above adults >50yo commonest form gen wrists & ankles if this involves a hairy region of the skin and the loss of hair follicules then it is also called...

Lichen Planopilaris AKA Acuminatus AKA Follicular lichen planus,AKA Lichen planus follicularis, AKA Peripilaris Lichen planopilaris is a distinct variant of Cicatricial Alopecia, a group of rare disorders which destroy the hair follicle, replace it with scar tissue, & cause permanent hair loss.

Aetiology autoimmune *see also* **Alopecia**

Lichen Simplex (chronicus) presents as a v itchy patch of thickened dry skin, which has exaggerated normal skin lines of long duration – or lesions - if cleared it will reappear.

Lichen Striatus presents as lines of skin bumps on one side of the body only - in children b/n 5-10 yo girls>boys. This is less itchy than other forms of Lichen, and may resolve completely.

Lichenification (Lī-ken-i-kay-shon) - an area of diffuse evenly raised thickening of the most superficial 3 strata of the skin - from S.Spinosum. Underlying lf. The skin has a mauvish leather-like appearance with exaggerated normal skin lines e.g. **Lichen simplex**

Lichenoid lichen-like – thickened skin lines, brawny colour thickened skin

Ligament. Lt ligate to tie (up) - sing. ligamentum pl ligamenta a band of tissue which connects bones (articular ligaments) or viscera - organs (visceral ligaments). A Ligament is a tie or a connection generally composed of collagen fibres.

Linea/linear a line as in the Nuchal lines of the Occiputum

Lingua *adj **Lingual*** pertaining to the tongue *see also* **Glossus**

Lipatrophy/lipodystrophy loss or changes in the subcut fatty tissue often assoc with other systemic disorders – *see also* **Panniculitis**

Lipoedema – abnormal accumulation of fat in the LL partic in women, may begin as cellulite, but progresses and does not involve the feet nor is the person necessarily obese or fat in other areas may lead to and be mistaken for Lymphoedema

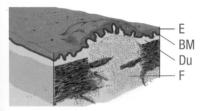

E
BM
Du
F

Lipoma benign tumour of fat cells presenting as a large smooth painless lump on the skin b/n 1/2-10cm **DD Epidermoid cysts**

Livedo (Liv-EE-doh) discoloured spot on the skin due to passive congestion –

    Post Mortem Livedo dark red congestion seen in post mortem colouration of the skin that shows the position of the death

Liver Spots *see* **Lentigo**

Livid *Lt **lividus** = **lead coloured*** discoloured from contusion or congestion

Locus (LOH-kus) a place - specific area in organ or tissue of either cell division or specialization

Lovibond angle – angle b/n the NF & the NP should be < 160^0 *see also* **Clubbing, MT NAILS – Nail plate abnormal shape**

-lucent (LOO-sent) transparent, clear

Lunula (Lun-OO-lah) the whitish proximal half moon shape at the base of the nail bed

Lupus (LOO-pus) *Lt = **wolf*** to depict a surface – generally skin which has a gnawed or eaten appearance

    Lupus Pernio is an unusual presentation of **Sarcoidosis** on the face – generally as purple plaque on the cheeks or nose *see* **Sarcoidosis**

Lupus Vulgaris presents as a slow-growing orange/red plaque on the face – is a presentation of tuberculosis In of the dermis **DD Birth mark**

Lyme disease is a tick borne disease
presents as a circular rash – Erythema Migrans – with enlarging target lesion on the limbs

-lymph (LIM-pf) clear liquid

Lymphangioma benign lesions that result only in a soft, slow-growing, "doughy" mass. generally in the neck **(AKA Cystic Hygroma)** but may occur anywhere which do not become malignant. Maybe congenital & assoc with chromosomal abnormalities

Aetiology malformation of lymphatics which result in abnormal drainage and fluid accumulation *see also* **Angiomas**

Lymphatic – a vessel which carries fluid – lymph - to the heart

Lymphocytes small round single nucleated WBCs derived from the BM or the thymus gld, one of the MNC types, which produce Abs and are involved in the IR *see also* **B cells, T cells**

Lymphokines Cytokines made by lymphocytes. *see also* **Cytokines, Interleukins**. All lymphokines are cytokines but not vv.

macro- big, large

Macrophage (MAK-roh-farj) Tissue MNC, originally from the BM to the BS & then migrated out to the T.

Macule a flat spot, non-palpable or patch on the skin of a different colour > 5mm e.g. freckles, lentigo *see also* **Lentigo**

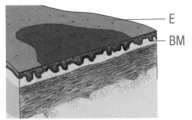

Madarosis – loss of eyelashes

Magnum *pl magna* large

Major histocompatibility complex (MHC) locus on cells to determine self & non-self

    Class I = found on all nucleated cells & present to Cytotoxic T cells

    Class II = found on certain immune cells B cells / Macrophages / dendritic cells – present to

    Helper T cells

Malar cheek

Malignant process which is rapid disconnected and uncontrolled as opposed to **benign** – so a malignant growth will be rapid and metastasize

Manuum hand

Mast cells large cells found in CTs throughout the body, most abundantly in the suBMucosal tissues & the dermis. They contain large granules which play a crucial role in allergic reactions *see also* **WBCs**

Measles a disease due to a viral In which has 10 days incubation before presenting on the skin with a red/purple rash & Koplik spots on the MM other SS are sore throat &cough, conjunctivitis, runny nose & tonsillitis

Melanin (MEL-an-in) pigment in melanocytes responsible for the main colouration of the skin & hair. There are 2 forms of melanin, the black, brown EUMELANIN and the yellow, red PHEOMELANIN. The amounts of each type is genetically determined *see also* **MT SKIN - pigmentation**

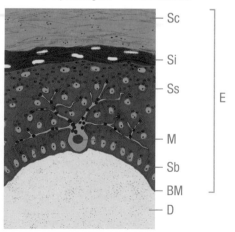

eumelanin   *pheomelanin*

Melanocyte (M) a cell of the epidermis responsible for its pigmentation – spreads branches b/n epidermal cells and disperses pigmented granules when stimulated – note is above the BM – if below this is pathological – *see* **Melanoma**

- Sc
- Si
- Ss
- M
- Sb
- BM
- D

E

Melanogenesis the formation of melanin

Melanoma a malignant growth of melanocytes from the base of the epithelial layer of the skin presents as an irregular poorly defined flat pigmented plaque or mole. It presents as an irregular poorly defined pigmented plaque or mole which enlarges. See ABCDE for a summary of changes indicative of melanoma (1) versus benign plaque or naevus (2)

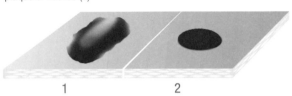

1   2

The melanocytes invade through the BM, move through the dermis and can spread via lymphatics or the BVs *see also* **Lentigo**

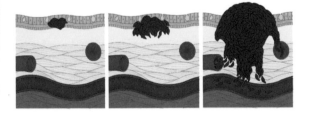

Acral Lentiginous Melanoma brown discolouration beneath the nail, palms or soles *see also* **MT NAILS**

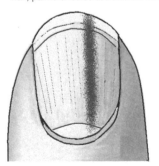

Melasma AKA the mask of pregnancy AKA Chloasma presents as dark pigmentation on the face of women who are pregnant or on Hormone Tx. May occur anywhere but the main sites are cheekbones around the mouth and the neck and chin.

Type of melasma	Clinical features
Epidermal	• well-defined border
	• dark brown
	• appears under black light
	• responds well to Tx
Dermal	• commonest
	• ill-defined border
	• light brown / bluish
	• too deep for black light
	• responds poorly to Tx
Mixed	• variegated colour with patches
	• mixed pattern under black light
	• partial improvement with Tx

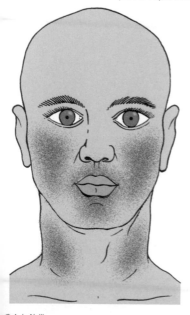

© A. L. Neill

Mentum *Lt chin* relating to the chin.

Merkel's cells AKA Merkel-Ranvier cells one of the many different sensory N endings in the skin assoc with light touch. The Merkel cell **(Mc)** senses changes in the keratinocytes **(E)** via desmosomes **(Ds)** which it feeds to the N cell **(N)** via granules **(G)** so generating an impulse – *see also* **MT SKIN epidermis**

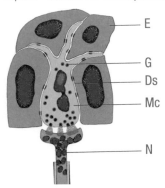

meta- an extension of... cf. metacarpal = extension of the wrist

Metaplasia the changing of one form of tissue type to another, extending from one type to another type as it grows

Micrographic surgery = Moh's technique – surgical technique used to excise lesions (L) mainly BCCs particularly the sclerosing type where the tumour is removed using a series of horizontal slices parallel to the skin's surface. The slices are taken deeper and deeper until the base limit of the tumour is cleared as determined by microscopy

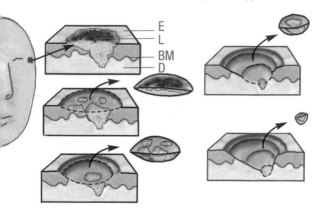

Microvasculature the network of small BVs arterioles ➡ capillaries ➡ venules in a tissue

Miliaria *Lt miliary – grainlike* **AKA Prickly Heat AKA Sweat rash AKA Heat rash** small itchy "prickly" red rash may be over large areas or more localized e.g. skin folds, axillae, head chest and neck

Aetiology blocked sweat glands -commoner in children as their sweat glands are underdeveloped, In with normal skin flora may precipitate or exacerbate the disease

Miliaria Crystalline – most superficial blockage appears as supf. blisters on the skin surface

Miliaria Rubra obstruction in the v deepest levels causing If and widespread erythema **DD Acne, Shingles** *see also* **Folliculitis**

Miliaria profunda most severe form often due to repeated episodes which get progessivleyl worse and more severe – clear coloured ill-defined rash widespread **DD Cellulitis**

Minoxidil is an antihypertensive vasodilator medication which also slows or stops hair loss & promotes hair re-growth partic. terminal hair *chemical name 6-piperidin-1-ylpyrimidine-2,4-diamine 3-oxide*

Mitosis (MY-toh-sis) *pl mitoses* normal cell division

Modiolus hub or central core used in the face to indicate that fibrous hub at the edge of the mouth for the insertion of a number of muscles / used in the ear to indicate the centre of the spongy bone of the cochlear tubes

Moh's technique *see* Micrographic surgery

Moisturisers AKA Emollients are complex compounds used to soften & hydrate the outer layers of the skin in partic – SCorneum.

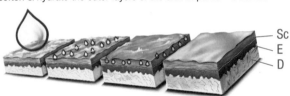

Sc
E
D

Common components are various light weight oils ± petroleum products ± aqueous creams – a mixture of oil and water based compounds with different emphases on each

3 mechanisms –

1 Occlusives to provide a thin layer to prevent evaporation from the surface

2 Humectants to attract moisture to the surface of the skin

3 Restorants – composed of chemicals deficient on the skin surface

Complications with application

1 blockage of the pore-water based s causing comedones

2 allergic reaction due to components and added fragrances etc

3 ln due to bacteria in the creams

4 possible ⬆ cancer because of components of the moisturizer

Uses

1 to maintain normal skin integrity – light weight oils

2 to moisten DRY skin (fissures)– heavier oils

3 to reduce OILY skin – water based substances – anticomedogenic

4 to relieve ichthyosis- itching / irritated skin / sensitive skin – calming oils – aqueous creams

5 ⬇ aging – oils with antioxidants

6 ⬇ flaking of psoriasis / eczema / erythema – aqueous creams light water based non-allergenic

Moisturizers are often included in sunscreens *see also* **Sunscreens**

Mole AKA Beauty spot, Birthmark, Naevus raised pigmented well demarcated overgrowth of epithelial cells. It is very common– the average person has about 10-20 moles.

Aetiology familial, sun exposure *see also* **Naevus**

Morbilliform rash – red /purple rash - similar to measles but w/o the systemic symptoms due to an enterovirus or drug reaction, which resolves after 2 days w/o residual effects

Molluscum contagiosum highly contagious tiny red - flesh coloured bumps on the skin in the genital area

Aetiology viral In

Mongolian spots AKA birthmarks blue-black marks on the lower buttocks of infants particularly of pigmented races, which often resolve.

Monocytes WBCs with a large single bean-shaped nucleus, part of the MNCs group. Monocytes that leave the BS are called macrophages & those residing in the T are histiocytes.

morph- (MORF-) shape / form

Morphea a purplish patch of skin, which thickens & becomes waxy white, then speckled discoloration. It may spontaneously resolve .

Aetiology unknown

Mosaicism (MOH-zay-ik-ism) AKA Chimera adj mosaic an individual demonstrating at least 2 sets of DNA origins, the pattern is a mosaic *see also* **Chimera**

Mucinosis abnormal deposits of mucin in the skin from fibrocytes often associated with Myxoedema (hypothyroidism)

Shar-Pei mucinosis associated with greatly increased wrinkled skin because of ⬆ deposits of mucin and so thickening and excessive dermal ground substance

Multiforme *see also* **Polymorphic**

myco- **(MY-coh)** relating to fungi

Myelocyte **(MY-loh-site)** – young cell in the WBC granulocyte series, may go on to become Acidophil, Basophil or Neutrophil.

Naevus AS Nevus (NEE-vus) *Lt birthmark pl naevi* any raised benign defect of the skin derived from cells of the skin, may be congenital or acquired most people have at least 1-10 by puberty and ⬆ with age

Course / Maturation – begin as flat macules which grow and elevate from the surface developing pigment until brown/black after which they slowly lose their pigment to become flesh coloured polymorphic polyps *see also* **Birthmark, Hamartoma, Cutaneous Hamartoma DD BCC, Lentigo, skin tags**

The Naevus is named via its site –

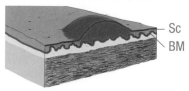

Sc
BM

superficial / junctional – when it is found solely in the epidermis

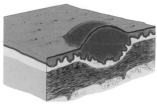

compound – when it is found in the epidermis & the dermis

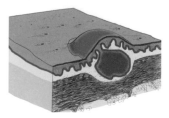

intradermal – when it is found only in the dermis and particular features as discussed below.

   Becker's Naevus demarcated hyperpigmented patch containing strong dark hairs

   Blue Naevus a harmless, dark-blue to grey-to-black, well defined spot or bump on the skin, from growth pigmented cells deep in the skin- melanocytes. Because these cells are deep in the skin the colour becomes blueish as it is seen through the other skin layers – when melanocytes are exposed on the surface of the skin they have a typical brown-black colour.

Types of these deep blue grey naevi include:

Ita's naevus – on the UL & shoulder

Ota's naevus – on the face partic around the eye (AKA **Hori's naevus**)

Dysplastic naevus acquired at adolescence & may take many forms **DD Melanoma**

Epidermal Naevus = Birthmark = Verricous epidermal naevus brown raised well demarcated variable size, warty appearance caused by aberrant keratocytes

Halo naevus raised mole with central pigmentation & pale surrounding tissue – due to IR to the Naevus so the lesion is attacked and pigment lost

Intradermal naevus skin coloured mole deep in the dermis so no pigmentation shows, stable, dome-shaped **DD BCC**, neurofibromas, skin tags

Melanocytic naevus AKA mole commonest form. It is composed of melanocytes

Naevus flammeus = Port wine stain = Angioma where the composite cell type is the capillaries - a vascular malformation generally on the face or neck which may increase and become nodular with age. *See also* **Angioma, Sturge-Weber syndrome**

Naevus sebaceous present from childhood with a yellowish warty surface & hair loss over their surface composed of cells from the sebaceous glands **DD BCC**

Nail-bed distal part of the finger / toe from which the nail grows

Nail- fungus *see* **Onychomycosis**

Nail-grooves grooves from b/n nail and skin surrounding the nail bed

Nail-plate hard square plate of the "nail"

Nappy Rash *see* **Dermatitis**

Nape AKA Nucha AKA scruff of the neck the posterior curve on the neck -

Naris nostrils *pl. Nares*

Necrosis (NEK-roh-sis) **GK necros death**, referring cell death, tissue death &/or organ death

Necrolysis death of cells due to liquification

Neoplastic (NEE-oh-plas-tik) *Gk neo = new plasia = growth* any uncontrolled growth which may metastasize and spread directly or indirectly in an uncontrolled or poorly controlled manner often losing many or all specialized features of their original tissue *see also* **Benign, Malignant**

Nests descriptive term for multiple cells orientated circularly and growing into the centre of the circle as opposed to cells with no particular orientation - **clusters**

Neurofibroma / Neurofibromatosis AKA Elephant man disease is an unusual hereditary disease of the skin and other organs). Typically it begins in childhood with multiple flat pigmented patches called *cafe-au-lait* spots, which become soft fleshy skin growths **neurofibromas.** *Most people that have solitary neurofibromas do not have neurofibromatosis.*

The disease neurofibromatosis involves bones, nerves & endocrine glands, but the extent varies.

Aetiology inherited dominant, idiopathic (for single lesions.

Course unpreditiable may progress to a serious fatal disease or remain as single lesions

Neutrophils AKA Granulocytes – WBCs with granular cytoplasm of neutral staining histologically & multi-lobed nuclei. When these migrate from the BS they are called polymorpho-nuclear cells (PMNs). *see also* **WBCs**

Nigricans darkening, a lesion which shows increased brown/black pigment

noci- (NOH-see) pain

Nodule adj nodular a lump deeply set in the skin > 5mm

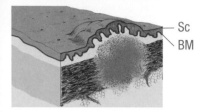

— Sc
— BM

Non-melanotic skin cancer (NMSC) skin cancer not derived from melanocytes. Because most skin cancers are melanomas – the rest are grouped in this fashion.

Nucha the nape or back of the neck *adj.- nuchal*

Nucleolus brain w/n the brain - nub of DNA material inside the nucleus

Nucleus nut – brain of the cell containing DNA

Nummular coin-like used to describe skin lesions which look like coins on the skin as in Nummular dermatitis

O'Briens granuloma = Actinic granuloma *see* **Granuloma**

Oedema AS Edema (uh-DEEM-uh) swollen *adj oedematous*

-oid like / similar to

-ology study of

-oma lump / tumour

Omo **(OH-moh)** shoulder

Ontogeny the development of an individual growth pattern

Onychauxis abnormal nail thickening w/o deformity due to systemic diseases

Onycho (on-EE-koh) pertaining to the nail

Onychocyte – nail producing keratinocytes

Onychogryphosis abnormal nail thickening due to P – generally the big toe crushed into ill-fitting shoes *see also* **NAILS**

Onychology the study of the nails & supporting structures

Onychomycosis a nail fungal In

Orf is a solitary 2cm growth on the fingers or hand. Initially a red growth – it becomes target shaped and crusts

    Aetiology contagious febrile viral In & assoc lymphadenopathy

Organelle one of the specialized parts of the protozoan or tissue cell

Orifice an opening.

ortho- straight

Orthokeratosis *see* **Keratosis**

-osis disease of – non-inflammatory

Ota's naevus *see* **Naevus**

Ovale oval shaped

Pachyonychia (PAK-ee-on-ik-ee-ah) *Gk paky = thick onyx = nail*
elephant nail – any abnormally thick nail

Paget's disease (of the Nipple) AKA Ductal carcinoma in situ (DCIS) AKA Intraductal carcinoma of the nipple

presents as a unilateral red scaly irritating plaque around one nipple. It has a long Hx and slowly enlarges presenting mainly in women > 50yo

Pallisading – term used to describe cells usually epithelial/epitheloid forming in lines like a fence around or along a structure

Palpebral pertaining to the eyelid

palpable – able to be felt upon examination

Panniculitis – an inflammatory layer in the D or Du of the skin

Histology - If cells may be found throughout the dermis (D) in a diffuse, lobar pattern or septal pattern (Sp) along the septal collagen fibres. There is often an associated vasculkitis

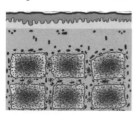 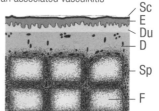

Sc
E
Du
D

Sp

F

e.g. Lobar panniculitis w/o vasculitis AKA acute panniculitis AKA systemic nodular pannicultis AKA Weber Christian disease.

SS tender skin nodules ± weight loss fatigue & other systemic symptoms

may present spontaneously after trauma e.g. cold exposure & spontaneously resolve – no systemic involvement

is assoc. with CT disorders; lymphoproliferative diseases; pancreatitis / pancreatic cancer, sarcoidosis

Panniculus *pl panniculi Lt pannus – garment / panniculus small garment* – layers or sheets of T covering organs in the body including the subcutaneous layer of fat just under the skin
panniculus adiposis

Panniculus adiposis AKA Subcutaneous fat AKA Superficial fascia

Panniculus carnosus – layer of striated muscle deep to the subcutaneous tissue which attached to the superficial fascia but no skeletal elements

Pannus AKA Granulation Tissue abnormal layer of fibrovascular T assoc with chronic IF - found in jts with Rheumatoid Arthritis, on the cornea & other areas. It contains If cells & substances - e.g. macrophages & interleukins which grow eroding & destroying the underlying tissue. It is always pathological.

Papilla – small budlike structure – in hair – the follicular dermal papilla (FDP)– cells from the dermis which induce the hair to grow *see* **Normal Hair section**

Papilloma *see* **Villoma**

Papule a raised spot on the skin's surface <5mm, small nodule. It may have a different colour (e.g. Lichen planus) ± scale – if it is generalized it is a **palpable rash** *see also* **Nodule**

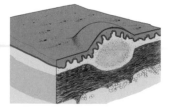

para- *Gk to one side*

Parakeratosis – immature SCorneum nuclei present, keratin, hence the skin is very dry & inflexible with oedema in the middle strata – the layers slough off easily & deep fissures may result. This is normal for cells of the MMs, which are in a moist environment *see also* **Keratosis**

Parietal *Lt paries, a wall* pertaining to the outer wall of a cavity

Paronychia (Pah-ron-IK-EE-uh) **AKA Whitlow** a bacterial In of the skin next to the nail. Signs of If - redness, swelling & pain are present, caused by a break in the nail to allow In.

Parotid pertaining to a region beside or near the ear

Pars a part of

Patch = large macule – non-palpable skin discolouration *see also* **Macule**

Pathergy phenomenon of scratching the skin slightly and causing lesions to develop – much like the Koebner phenomenon seen in **Behcert's disease & Pyoderma gangrenosum**

Pathogenesis the origin or cause of the pathology of a disease.

Pathogens MOs / substances that can cause disease when they infect/invade a host.

Pathophysiology the part of the science of disease concerned with disordered function as distinguished from physical defects.

-pathy disease of

Pediculosis capitis AKA head lice AKA Nits.

SS itchy red lumps on the scalp of children with "moving white flakes – which are lice and small white balls attached to the hair shafts – lice eggs. It is very contagious.

Pedis pertaining to feet

Pellagra (the 4 Ds) dermatitis (photodermatits), diarrhea, dementia, death

Aetiology niacin defic

Pemphigus *Gk pemphix = blister adj pemphigoid* group of skin diseases distinguished by recurrent crops of vesicles & bullae which often leave severe residual scarring. They are not contagious

Aetiology AI

Bullous Pemphigoid blisters on the MMs, may be due to reaction of the diet.

Cicatricial Pemphigoid blistering on the MMs around the eye, on the ocular conjunctiva

Pemphigus Foliaceus abundant small fragile superficial blisters on skin areas which break leaving a scaly red skin **DD Lupus erythematosis**

-penia (PEEN ee-yuh) lack of

peri- around

Perikymata transverse ridges & the grooves on the surfaces of teeth

Perivascular surrounding BVs generally capillaries

Perlèche AKA Cheilosis AKA Angular Stomatitis presents as a moist, red or white In b/n the skin folds at the corners of the mouth. There may be cracks or fissures & often it is sore or tender.

Aetiology – Vitamin B ± Zn deficiency with 2° yeast or other fungal In of the corners of the lips

hypervitaminosis A
poorly set false teeth &/or mouth closure in the elderly
2° anorexia / bulimia / poor nutrition

Perma- lines – AKA Wrinkles that are present all the time (as opposed to transient wrinkles which change with expressions)

Perniosis *adj Pernio* doughy subcutaneous swelling as seen in **Chilblains** *see also* **Chilblains**

Petechia (e) (per-TEEK-ee-uh) small <3mm

 red or purple spot on the body, caused by a minor haemorrhage – broken capillary BV. Used to describe the appearance of purpuric rashes, & may be caused by trauma or excessive P, or may be due to thrombocytopaenia - non blanchable.

pH a logarithmic measure of the amount of free H+ ions in solution determining the acidity or otherwise, generally b/n 0 -14 with 7 being neutral. Common pH levels – sebum, skin 4.5 - 5.5, most shampoos & soap 9-10

phaeo- (FAY-oh) brown dusky

phago- (FAY-goh) to eat / eater

Phagocyte any cell that can ingest/eat bacteria, foreign particles, &/or other cells.

-phil (FILL) lover of

Phimosis (FIM-oh-sis) *Gk phimos = muzzle* tight foreskin – which stops full retraction of the glans penis,

Phlegmon (FLEG-mon) unconfined If – as opposed to **Abscess** confined If *see also* **Cellulitis**

-phobe (FOBE) hater of

photo- to do with the sun

Photodistribution description of a skin lesion affected by exposure to the sun e.g. sunburn

Photoonycholysis lifting of the nail from it NB when exposed to the sun – as in tetracycline administration

Pilar pertaining to the hair

pilo- pertaining to hair *see also* **Tricho-**

Pilo-Sebaceous Unit Hair follicle + associated appocrine and sebaceous glands used to nourish the growing hair *see also* **Sebaceous**

Pimples *see* **Pustules**

Pityriasis (pit-EE-rï-a-sis) *Gk pityea = bran* any flaking of the skin

Pityriasis Alba presents as light coloured patches of skin of young adults & children located on the face, arms & trunk, asymptomatic

Aetiology In, familial , melanocytes not delivering pigment to the keratinocytes (may itch) **DD Vitiligo**

Pityriasis Amiantacea AKA Tinea amiantaceais (amiantaceus = asbestos-like) is a scaly thick white dermatitis of the Scalp resulting in hair loss because of the tightly adherent scales **DD Psoriasis, Seborrheaic Dermatitis Lichen Planus**

Pityriasis Capitus *see* **Dandruff, Dermatitis**

Pityriasis Rosea presents on young adults, as an oval, slightly scaly patch (called the herald patch) which up to 6 weeks later forms multiple smaller itchy patches. It appears to be a viral In **DD Tinea**

Plaque (plark) a raised uniform thickening of a portion of skin with a well defined edge and either a flat or rough surface e.g. **Psoriasis**

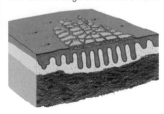

Plasma cells – derived from B cells are large Ab producing cells with central clock-faced nuclei

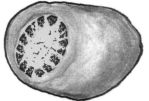

-plasia (PLAY-zee-uh) growth

-podia (POH-dee-uh) pertaining to feet (often the formation of feet for cell movement)

poikilo- spotted, mottled, irregular

poly- many

Polymorphic many shaped see also Multiforme

Polymorphic light eruption appears hrs after UV exposure as itchy red papules vesicles or plaques which last for days & then resolves as the patient develops tolerance for the UV / sun exposure *see also* **Sunburn**

Polyp (PO-lip) - a small stalk-like protrusion of tissue that grows out of the membranes lining various areas of the body including skin common on various MMs e.g. nasal polyps *see also* **Acrochordon, Skin tags**

Polythrichia - excessive hair growth often regional

Pompholyx (POM-fo-liks) = Dyshidrotic Eczema presents as tiny water blisters localized to the hands & feet, which erupt causing a scaly eruption on the palms & sides of the fingers, with intense itching

Porphyria (POR-free-yuh) *Gk = blue pigment* – series of diseases where the precursors to produce haemoglobin – porphyrins - accumulate in the skin & body, due to enzyme abnormalities, presents with dark coloured urine

> **Porphyria cutanea tarda** appears as blisters & small white bumps on the back of the hands & the face. The skin is fragile, photosensitive & easily injured. The face grows extra hair & develops dark areas of discoloration around the eyes.
>
> Aetiology familial, iatrogenic, adverse drug reaction

Port wine stain *see also* **Naevus Flammeus, Angioma** presents as a reddish purple vascular birthmark of the skin, occurring unilaterally – generally on the face - blanchable

Prickle cells AKA spinocytes, cells of the SSpinosum

Primula poison of primrose which like poison ivy causes severe swelling & redness of the skin in sensitive subjects

Process a general term describing any marked projection or prominence as in the mandibular process.

Pro-inflammatory cytokines family of cytokines that promote If. e.g. TNF = tumor necrosis factor

Prominens a projection

Proximal closer to the axial skeleton (opposite of **Distal**)

Prickly Heat *see* **Miliaria**

Pruritis (PROO-ri-tis) *Lt = itch* the urge to itch

  Pruritis Ani AKA Anusitis – urge to scratch the anus

pseudo- false

Pseudofolliculitis AKA Shave bumps AKA Ingrown hairs presents as red bumps, ingrown hairs, or pus bumps on the beard area of the face & neck.- the hair is cut below the skin and grows inwards piercing the hair pore and causing If. Commoner in curly hair.

Psoriasis (SAW-rri-a-sis) = Psoriais vulgaris is a chronic recurring disease an autoimmune familial skin disease. Due to an IR signals are sent to the skin ± its adnexae to speed up the growth cycle, partic of the upper layers, causing deposition of excessive scales on the epidermal surface. Its distinguishing feature is the silver scale (Si) on the multiple, red, well defined, thickened skin lesions, and it may have spongiform features (sp), with or w/o purulent invasion by PMNs. It is associated with arthritis partic of the finger & toe jts, nail changes & stroke, *see also* **Koebner phenomenon**

severity is determined by the PASI = psoriatic area severity index – proportional to the skin coverage (0-72)

  Aetiology Alm, familial, post infective in susceptible people

  5 types are recognized

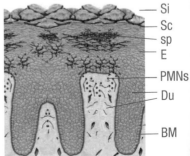

Si
Sc
sp
E
PMNs
Du
BM

© A. L. Neill

Erythrodermic plaques more inflamed

Guttate Psoriasis appears as multiple, small, red, teardrop shaped scaly bumps which suddenly appear on the trunk, arms & legs. It may be preceded by a sore throat & a cold generally from a Streptococcal In.

Inverse / flexural smooth plaques on flexural surfaces, in skin folds & under an overweight abdomen (Panniculus) or breasts.

Plaque Psoriasis elbows & knees present with snowy, silvery plaques

Psoriatic nail dystrophy together with other sites or isolated nail changes including yellowing, pitting & onycholysis

Pustular Psoriaris pus filled plaques generally on the hands & feet, PMNs + T cell involvement assoc with spongiform changes

DD Eczema, dermatitis – plaques here are on the inside of the jt

Psoriaform hyperplasia – description of changes to epidermis in Psoriasis

Pterygium (TER-rij-ee-um) wing

Pubis (PEW-bis) hairy that part of the hip bone with hair over the surface *adj pubic pl pubes*

Puritis *see* **Itching** note this term is used as a shortening of Puritis Ani – itch of the anus

Purpura (PER-PER-ruh) = *Lt purple* a rash which is due to a vasculitis or bleeding into the dermis - 3 forms those > 3mm in diameter those < 3mm diameter – does not blanch with pressure *see also* **Petechiae**

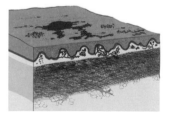

Schamberg's purpura AKA Pigmented Purpuric Dermatosis presents as tiny red unblanchable spots on the legs, which degenerate to yellow-brown spots before resolving.- months later. Due to the increased P on the legs with poor venous return &/or oedema the B is forced from the capillaries into the skin

Solar Purpura AKA Actinic purpura AKA senile purpura is a common condition of elderly skin, which has lost a lot of strength & integrity– shearing b/n the layers results in bleeding into the tissue

Pus purulent fluid of AIF composed of PMNs & necritic material

Pustule = Pimple a skin bleb filled with pus (P) or purulent fluid *see also* **Acne, Spongiform**

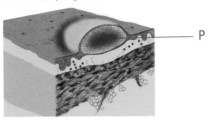

pyo- (Pĭ-oh) *Gk pus*

Pyoderma (Pĭ-OH-derm-uh) *adj pyogenic* any purulent skin disease
   Impetago
   Pyoderma gangrenosum

Pyogenic Granuloma presents as a well defined raised red or violaceous lump on the skin that may easily bleed, multiple & recurring it is self limiting **DD BCC** *see also* **Granuloma**

Quick = Hyponychium

Rash a change of the skin which affects its color, appearance &/or texture – multiple lesions close together. It may be localized or generalized & is often associated with an AR, IR &/or IfR - may be blanchable or purpuric

Morbilliform rash - a rash which looks like measles

Raynaud's phenomenon overreactive vasospastic disorder in the extremities fingers / toes – BVs contract in cold and cause hypoxia in these areas – hence wasting & deterioration - in extreme conditions death of the digits etc will result. The skin turns pale cyanotic and later swells and reddens with parasthesia **DD Scleroderma**

Rectus (REK-tus) *AKA ortho* straight - erect

recte- straight

rete ridges deep epidermal ridges which dip into the dermis & increase the surface area – the upward projections from the dermis are the dermal papillae. These are particularly deep in the volar & solar surfaces, *see* **SKIN - dermis.**

Reticular net-like pattern

Rhinus/rhino- pertaining to the nose

Rhinophyma (RY-no-Fī-muh) presents as a bulbous enlargement of the nose (men) due to hyperplasia of the regional sebaceous glands associated with **Rosacea** – not associated with alcohol

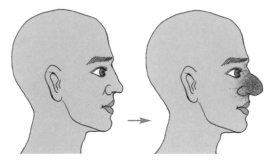

Ridge elevated growth often roughened

Ringworm = Tinea Capitus, Tinea Corporis AKA Kerion

Rodent Ulcer a BCC with a central ulceration, highly invasive often causing a lot of local T destruction *see also* **BCC**

Rosacea (ROHZ-say-SHEE-uh) presents on the face and cheeks in adults >30yo usually with fair skin – longstanding cases lead to thickened skin (partic on the nose) & telangiectasia *see also* **Rhinophyma, SLE**

	ACNE	ROSECEA
SYMPTOMS	• Pimples • Whiteheads • Blackheads • Inflammation	• Redness in center of face • Nose enlargement • Pimples • Itching
CAUSE	• Plugged pores • Infection in pores • Ingrown hairs • Hormone changes • Always involves the HF	• Weather change ⬆ wind ⬆ heat • Emotional stress • Alcohol consumption • Reaction to germs and other content of the pores • Reaction to makeup/ skin care products • Always involves the skin BVs
VULNERABLE INDIVIDUALS	• Most commony teens • Adult women, on chin and jaws • Adult men, on backs	• Adults over 30 • Women more than men • Fair-skinned people

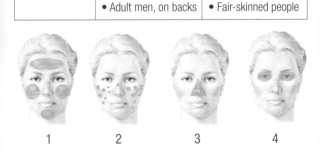

1   2   3   4

There are 4 main subtypes of rosacea

1. persistant facial flushing
2. "bumps, "pimples", raised patches on the face
3. enlarged nose (♂ > ♀ rhinphyma)
4. persistant eye redness

Roseola Infantum AKA Sixth disease commonest form of pink/red rash in infants no other SS are present lasts 2-3 days resolves completely **DD Rubella**

Rubella AKA German Measles is a viral disease which incubates for 14-21 days before a light pink rash appears spreading for 24hrs then fading. LNs are swollen and there may be joint pain. This disease is only of significance because of its effect on the unborn foetus. If infected in the 1st trimester the mother may give birth to a severely affected baby.

Rubelliform like Rubella – light pink rash as opposed to **mobilliform rash** which is measle-like – smaller, redder spots

Salmon patch AKA Capillary Angioma *see* **Angioma**

Sarcoid (SAR-koyd) *Gk sarc -flesh* *see also* **Granulomas**

Sarcoidosis a disease in which "sarcoid deposits " resembling granulomas are placed in various organs in the body including in 25% of cases the skin. In the skin the disease is self limiting, but the disease may resolve spontaneously or continue and prove fatal it is difficult to Dx and treat.

Aetiology idiopathic *see also* **Granulomatosis**

Sarcoma – *Gk fleshy lump* malignant tumour derived from cells of mesenchymal (CT) origin

Scabies AKA itch mite an highly infectious skin condition caused by ***Sarcoptes scabiei****.* a tiny mite (around 0.2-0.4mm) which burrows into the skin and causes red bumps & intense itching 4 weeks later. It is spread through: direct skin contact with an infected person & by contaminated bedding, towels & clothes. Presents as fine blueish grey lines in skin folds & or genitals partic in males, but may appear anywhere generally not on the face or scalp.

Mites may live for days away from the host so it is difficult to eradicate (animal equivalent is **Mange** but this is due to a different mite species) *see also* **Burrows**

Scalded skin syndrome *see* **Bullous Impetigo**

Scale a flake of flat horny cells – loosened from the horny layer (SCorneum) often assoc with parakeratosis **e.g. Parakeratosis, Psoriasis**

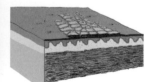 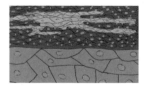

Sebaceous cyst blocked skin pores lead to a build up of sebum in the HS. If this becomes infected it leads to acne, if not it forms a sebaceous cyst, which may or may not involve a hair

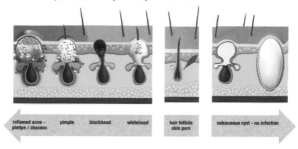

inflamed acne -   pimple   blackhead   whitehead   hair follicle   sebaceous cyst - no infection
pimlpe / abscess   skin pore

Scalene uneven

Scar *see also* **Keloid** the result of healing of an ulcer – full skin defect – where the skin is replaced with fibrous T & the epithelial specializations are lost.

   hypertrophic scar this occurs when the CT is raised above the skin line & appears hard - if it extends beyond the area of Iy, it is a **Keloid**

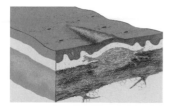

Scarlet Fever *β haemolytic Strep* In, presents as sore throat, lymphadenopathy, anorexia, scarlet tongue with enlarged papillae (strawberry tongue) then a bright red rash. It is highly contagious

Schamberg's purpura AKA pigmented purpuric dermatosis *see* **Purpura**

Sclersosis hard / hardening *adj sclerotic*

Scleroderma AKA Systemic Sclerosis hardening of T & organs

in skin hardening of the skin with tightening of the surface itching and dermal and muscle wastage

Scoring systems in dermatology – *see* **MT SKIN**

Scoring systems in dermatology – There are several systems in dermatology to determine on a quasi-quantitative scale the severity of a disease e.g. eczema and allow for inter and intra-patient comparison.

Scurvy – *Lt Scorbitus = ascorbic acid adj scorbutic*

AKA Barlow's disease when in infants

Presentation red non-blanchable skin spots, easy bruising, poor wound healing, malaise & lethargy, bone pain, bleeding gums & loose teeth

Aetiology deficiency in Vitamin C

Pathogenesis the inability to stabilize collagen which is constantly turned over and needed in skin, MM & all CT maintenance & wound healing

see also **Diseases of Micronutrient deficiency – Beriberi, Pellagra**

Sebum wax / oily substance *adj sebaceous*

Sebaceous cysts – *see* **Cyst**

Seborrhoeic *AS Seborrheic*

Seborrhoeic Dermatitis AKA Dandruff AKA Pityriasis Capitis see **Dermatitis** scaly uninflamed rash on hair bearing areas with loose white flakes

Aetiology In of normal skin yeast – Malassezia / Pityrosporum ovale **DD Psoriasis**

Seborrheic keratosis AKA Age Spots *see* **Keratosis**

Sebum wax / oily substance secreted by the sebaceous glands *adj sebaceous* pH is generally b/n 4.5 -5.5 and part of the acid mantle of the skin and essential to the health and flexibility of the hair.

Selective Photothermolysis AKA Laser treatment is the process of delivering energy to selectively destroy the desired target, which could be hair, pigment or tattoo dye etc. Factors to be selected for the specific target are: fluence (radiant exposure), pulse duration & wavelength. The laser's energy heats the target above the necrotic temperature but the duration is such that surrounding T is not affected. Generally thick coarse hairs can take longer lower pulse durations which are ineffective on finer hairs.

The depth of the laser penetration **(L)** will determine the target. Some of the uses are shown below.

Shallower pulses will target pigments in the Melanocytes **(M)** to reduce age spots etc., the sebaceous glands for Acne **(A)**, deep into the dermis to remove dermal pigments **(P)** as in tattoos, the hair roots to explode the follicules **(H)** for hair removal, deeper for BVs to remove telangiectasia formation, and as deep as the deep fascial layers **(F)** for skin tightening and fat removal

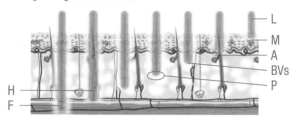

Senile old

Serpiginous snake-like, creeping e.g. to describe a burrowing pattern under the skin by an MO – describes lesions which scar the T below the skin surface while affecting the top layers *see also* **Tinea**

Serratus serrated, saw-toothed

Sesamoid grainlike

Shingles *see* **Herpes Zoster Varicella**

Sigmoid S-shaped, from the letter Sigma which is S in Greek.

Sinus a space usually w/n a bone lined with MM, such as the frontal & maxillary sinuses in the head, (also, a modified BV usually vein with an enlarged lumen for blood storage & containing no or little muscle in its wall). Sinuses may contain air, venous or arterial blood, lymph or serous fluid depending upon location and health of the subject *adj.- sinusoid*.

In the skin it is a canal linking the subcut T or deeper with the outside – and may weep fluid and be difficult to heal

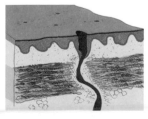

Sjörgens syndrome (SHOH-grins) autoimmune disease present in women > 40 where the cells attack the exocrine glands – and cause: dryness of the eyes, xerophthalmia; mouth, xerostoma & other MMs including; conjunctiva, keratoconjunctivitis sicca, and other areas nose,skin, vagina etc collectively referred to as SICCA symptoms. It is assoc with RA and other AI diseases.

Skin tag = Fibroepithelial polyp = Acrochordon DD Mole *see also* **Polyp**

Solar referring to the sun – used to indicate a cause of the skin change *see also* **Actinic**

Solar Elastosis *see* **Elastosis**

Solar Purpura AKA Actinic Purpura AKA Senile Purpura *see* **Purpura.**

Sore (SAW) *see* **Ulcer**

Sore mouth *see* **Orf**

SPF sun protection factor a measure of the effectiveness of sunscreens in preventing exposure to sunlight in particular to the UVB – the Ultraviolet light which causes sunburn.

The factor refers to the increase as a multiple in the time the person can be exposed to the sun (at full strength) as would be experienced w/o any sunscreen. Hence SPF15 indicates the person can be exposed 15X as long to the sun. However this does not take into account the cream wearing off or the sun's strength altering. Note also unless specified the SPF refers only to UVB

see also **Sunscreens**

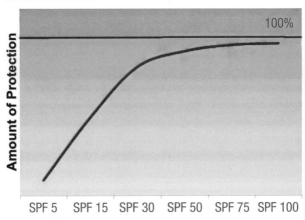

© A. L. Neill

Spider Angiomas AKA **Spider Telangiectasia** AKA **Vascular Spiders** AKA **Spider Naevi** *see* **Angioma** present as a network of capillaries on the skin with a central enlarged spot and "legs" coming out -which blanch on P *see also* **Telangiectasia**

Spine a thorn ***adj. - spinous*** descriptive of a sharp, slender process/protrusion

Spinocyte AKA **Prickle cell** – keratinocyte which is in SSpinosum

Split ends *see* **Trichoptilosis**

Spongiosis *adj spongiform* inter-epithelial swelling - inter-epithelial oedema

swelling may be due to serous exudates b/n epithelial cells

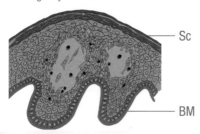

or it may be purulent – i.e. filled with pus – AKA **Munro's microabscesses** also seen in **Psoriasis & Seborrheaic dermatitis**

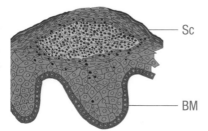

Sporotrichosis is a fungal skin In of the hand or finger. A growth under the skin may appear at the site of In or it may be an open sore. Nodules may grow advancing up the arm. There can be considerable swelling of the fingers, hand and arms. It is caused by ***Sporotrix schenckii*** a fungus found in the soil. Gardeners, horticulturists, florists, landscapers are at risk for the condition

Squamous flat, square-shaped *see* **Epithelial cells**

Squamous cell carcinoma (SCC) skin cancer derived from squamous epithelial cells - may occur wherever there is an epithelial layer and take many forms. Distinguishing features the hard irregular edge **(ed)** and the epithelial cells breaking through the BM **(n)** to directly invade tissues - can break off and metastasize, often has a central necrotic area **(C)** May present as a painless red ulcer.

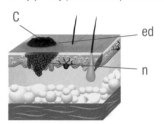

Stasis dermatitis *see* **Dermatitis**

Steven Johnson syndrome AKA Toxic Epidermal Necrolysis *see* **Erythema Multiforme Major**

Steroid is a type of organic compound that contains a characteristic arrangement of four cyclo-alkaline rings that are joined to each other. The commonest steroid in the body is cholesterol (C) from which all steroid Hs including cortisol (CL), the oestrogens (O) and the androgens (A) are derived.

Steroid Facies AKA Moon face resulting reversible red rash ± blisters with **Telangectasia** on cheeks due to application of topical steroids or ingestion of oral steroids, wide fat face & neck, which extends to the trunk, may also have increased facial hair, SLE **DD Rosacea**

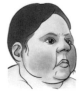

Stoma mouth

Strand as in strand of hair – a single hair

Stratified layered

Stratum sheet-like mass of substance / layer / lamina *pl strata*

Stratum adamantium dental enamel

Stratum basale epidermidis (Sb) = Basal stratum / base layer (of the skin) sits on the BM and divides to provide the cells for the other skin layers

Stratum corneum (Sc) outer horny/keratinized layer of the skin (dead cells)

Stratum corneum unguis outer horny layer of the nail = nail plate

Stratum granulosum (Sg) cells with nuclei, & accumulating keratin granules

Stratum germinativum = Sb + Ss
  = keratinocytes in the hair follicle which form the HS

Stratum lucidum (SL) = just under the Sc clear dead cells filled with keratin granules

Stratum malphigii (Sm) = Ss + Sg

Stratum spinosum (Ss) spiny layer of epithelial cell in the epidermis *see* **MT SKIN - epidermis**

Stria *pl striae adj striate* (Stry-u; – Stry-EE; Stry-ate) stripe

Striae AKA Stretch marks common acquired condition of the skin, presents as parallel bands of discoloration on the skin, associated with growth spurts or rapid weight gain, as in pregnancy. Initially bright red or deep purple they gradually fade to atrophic white bands which are permanent. When forming they may itch but are often asymptomatic, & they thin & weaken the epidermis (E), reduce the depth and number of dermal papillae (P) & places the collagen closer to the surface (Sc), forming a separation b/n the skin with dermal papillae & the thinner stretched striae (S).

Striae Gravidarum – stretch marks of pregnancy often with a single midline striae Linea Nigra **(LN)**

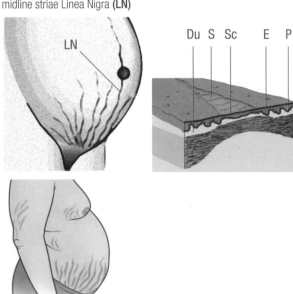

© A. L. Neill

Stroma (STROH-muh) *adj stromal* background tissue which may be fibrillar with occasional resident cells present, or matrix & extracellular material, in a tissue, ground substance and the associated cells present which do not represent the main tissue or organ support

Sturge-Weber syndrome a BV malformation present from birth involving the face ocular tissue ± the brain T – CNV_1 resulting in severe complications – **a severe Port-Wine stain** *see also* **Angioma**

Stucco hardening

Stye *see* **Hordeolum**

sudo- pertaining to sweat

Subcutus adj subcutaneous literally under the skin (the cutis) term used to define subcutaneous fat region below the hypodermis, in some cases used interchangeably with hypodermis which is the part of the dermis which lies below the thick collagen bands *see* **Hypodermis**

Subungal under the nail *see also* **Hyponychium**

Subunguis AKA Soleplate – modified epithelium under the nail plate or unguis

Sulcus furrow

Sun Spots AKA Actinic Keratoses *see* **Keratosis**

Sunburn after sun exposure the skin will present with erythema, swelling pain, and later develop blisters crusts & "peeling" soft skin e.g. eyelids etc are v sensitive *see also* **Sunscreens**

Sunscreens generally refer to creams, lotions and other materials applied to the skin's surface. Some of which act as barriers to the UV - physical sunscreens (PS) - reflecting the light, while others absorb the UV - chemical sunscreens (CS). Not all sunscreens block UVA (A) which has a shallower penetration than UVB (B). *See also* **SPF, Tanning, UV.**

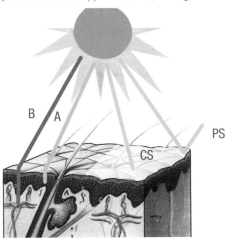

Superior above

Suppuration *adj suppurating see also* **pus**

Sycosis (SY-koh-sis) Chronic If of hair follicules, especially of the beard, with suppuration.

    herpetic sycosis Herpes In of the beard area
    lupoid sycosis – scarring form of deep folliculitis
    tinea barbae AKA Barber's itch ringworm of the beard

Syn- (SIN) means together ie the close proximity of or fusion of 2 structures.

Syringoma(s) sweat gland tumours 1-3 mm flesh coloured – axilla, eye lid, umbilicus and vulval areas **DD Xanthelasma.**

Systemic involving the whole body

Systemic Lupus erythematosis SLE an autoimmune, chronic If, relapsing, remitting disease. SLE can affect any organ system, but mainly involves the skin, joints, kidneys, blood cells, & NS. Ab/Ag complexes are placed on the BM of the skin and kidneys has a characteristic butterfly rash on the face similar to Rosacea.

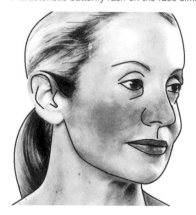

T cells = T lymphocytes 1 of the 2 major types of lymphocyte. These cells have sub groups but all are derived from the thymus. Reduction in these numbers results in reduced immune protection and excess may cause AI diseases.

Tanning – the increased brown pigmentation in the skin caused by UV stimulation. UVA causes increased release of melanin to the keratinocytes. UVB caused increased synthesis of melanin in the melanocytes. *See also* **Sunburn**

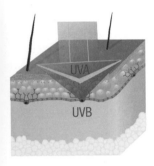

Targetoid target-like, circular with concentric rings

Tattoo foreign dye material in the dermis ingested by resident macrophages remains in the area and marks the skin

- taxis locomotor movement of cells

Telangectasia AKA Angioectasias (T) permanent dilatation of pre-existing capillaries generally smaller than angiomas generally they fill from the periphery. If they fill from the centre – **Spider angiomas (SA) = Spider Telangectasias** *see also* **Angioma**

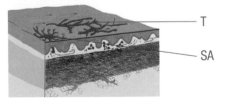

© A. L. Neill

Teledermatology sub-specialty of dermatology where images are sent distances to the specialist for evaluation – this is partic suited for dermatology as skin diseases are partic visible & in most cases do not need intrusive measure for assessment – it is to be noted the large numbers of helpful dermatological sites which can be used by all for ref in Dx of skin conditions

Telogen part of the normal hair growth cycle – long slow growing stage *see* **MT HAIR**

Temporal refers to time and the fact that grey hair (marking the passage of time) often appears first at the site of the temporal bone, from the consideration of wisdom in the temple.

Tendon a tie or cord of collagen fibres connecting muscle with bone (as opposed to articular ligaments which connect bone with bone)

Thrombocyte AKA Platelet – small piece of a megakaryocyte which circulates in the B to plug up any damage in the BVs and stimulate the clotting process

Thrombophlebitis an inflammatory swelling of the vein due to blood clots, may cause skin rupture and is painful partic in the LL.

Tight junctions AKA Tight junctional complex (TJC) formation of membrane-membrane fibrillar connections b/n cells for increased intercellular communication and strength consists of ZO & ZA *see also* **Desmosome**

Tinea (tin-EE-ya) AKA Ringworm a localized fungal infection due to a number of different fungi in susceptible patients with reduced immune system

> **Tinea corporis** is a fungal In of the skin that can occur at any age. It presents as a large, red, ring shaped itchy rash on the skin, with normal skin in the centre as the fungi eats the keratin in the outgrowing skin. Ringworm can occur anywhere on the skin. It is contagious & can be "caught" from many sources, including pets.

> **Tinea cruris AKA Jock Itch** occurs in the groin exacerbated by sweat and so is common in athletes

> **Tinea Manum AKA hand fungus** occurs on the hand, presents as a scaly, rash on the palms of the hands & b/n the fingers.

> **Tinea Pedis AKA athlete's foot** occurs on the feet/ foot of athletes because of the increased sweating with exercise

> **Tinea Unguium** occurs on the nails – big toe especially

Tinea versicolour AKA Sun Spots presents as well defined pale regions on the skin exacerbated after sun exposure. It is common and caused by a superficial yeast In on the skin surface. of people with compromised immune systems. The yeast organism is present on all skins but only present in suspecpuble people – the yeast organism blocks the formation of skin pigment (melanin) and the results may last for weeks or years

TNM staging of skin tumors replaces the older staging of melanomas

> **T** = tumor – tumor thickness in mm +
> a = no ulceration / b = ulceration
>
> **N** = node – number of LNs involved
>
> **M** = metastasis- number indicating distant spread of the tumor number looks like T1aN0M0 = tumor 1mm thick no ulcer no nodal involvement & no metastases

Toner AKA Skin fresheners AKA Astringents - imprecise term used to indicate a substance which cleans, "refreshes" & "tightens" the pores on the skin. Most of these substances are humectant moisturizers with varying amounts of alcohol content. They are not suitable for dry skin & are generally used in conjunction with other less stimulating moisturizers applied after the toner has dried or been removed, *see also* **Cleansers, Moisturizers**

Totalis – in an overall area as opposed to a localized area

Toxic poisonous

Toxic Epidermal Necrolysis AKA Steven Johnson syndrome *see* **Erythema Multiforme Major**

Transverse to go across

Trichiasis abnormally growing eyelashes – may grow back and scratch the cornea causing irritation – or growing from the medial canthus or naso fold into the eye

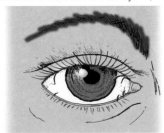

　　　　　　　　　© A. L. Neill

tricho- *Gk thrix = hair*

Trichotillomania a disorder where the sufferer pulls out their hair – including: eyelashes, eyebrows etc

Trichosis / Trichopathy any disease of the hair including abnormal growth *see also* **Hirsuitism**

Trichorrhexis AKA Split ends is a defect in the hair shaft characterized by thickening or weak points (nodes) that cause the hair to break off easily or split

Tricophyton fungus that generally causes athlete's foot, & ringworm

Trichoptilosis (TRIK-oh-til-oh-sis) AKA Split ends a longitudinal splitting of the hair fibre.

Trigone triangle

Trunk generally refers to the abdominal region not including the chest *see also* **Corp**

Tubercle a small process or bump, an eminence

Tumor AS Tumour lump, swelling

Tumour Necrosis factor (TNF) family of cytokines first implicated in cancers causing cell death, known to be involved in the IfR

Tylosis symmetric thickened scaly hyper-pigmented plaques on the palms ± the soles strongly associated with oesophageal carcinoma & assoc with Psoriasis

Ulcer – *Lt Ulcus adj ulcerated, ulcerative* an area of total loss of the epithelium from the skin or MM, a defect **AKA Sore**

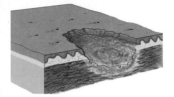

Unguis AKA nail plate

Unguium AKA fungal nail infection AKA Onychomycosis *see* **Tinea**

Universalis *see* **Totalis**

Urticaria (ER-tee-kair-ree-uh) *adj urticarial* vascular dilatation of BVs in the upper dermis usually transient, associated with wheals & preceded by intense itching, appears as red raised smooth papules. It also appears to be an AR to many varied & sometimes unknown stimuli *see also* **Hives**

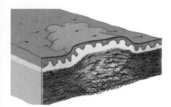

UV = ultra violet light *Lt beyond violet* as this is the last visible colour before UV range

This light is beyond the human visible range of light. The most important UVs in skin care are UVA & UVB and because of the ⬆ exposure to sterilizing equip UVC which otherwise is almost completely filtered by the ozone layer.

used to sterilize equipment

see **Chart on next page.**

see also **Sunscreens**

UV type	Wavelength range (nm)	Energy / photon (e-V)	effects	features
A = long wave (black light)	400-315	3.1-4.0	↑melanin release – quick tan ↑destruction of collagen fibres –(↑aging) ↑Vita A & D in the skin can form a Wood's light	98% of all UV board band sunscreen needed for protection glass is no protection, plastic acts as a barrier
B = medium wave	315-280	4.0-4.4	↑melanin synthesis – long lasting tan ↑sunburn ↑destruction of collagen fibres –(↑aging) ↑DNA + damage ↓Vita D ↑Vita A	all sunscreens block this glass acts as a barrier
C = short wave (germicidal)	280-100	4.4-12.4	↑DNA ++ damage	<.1% of the UV in atmosphere all sunscreens are effective, glass acts as a barrier, used in bug zapper lights used to sterilize equipment

Varicella AKA Herpes Zoster AKA Chicken pox

variegate patterned

Vasculitis If of the BVs – wrt as red, swollen painful skin

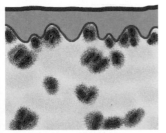

Varix *adj Varicose* – dilated as in varicose veins

Venerial warts *see* **Chodyloma Accuminata**

Verruca = Veruga = wart lobulated hyperplastic epidermal lesion, may be caused by the papilloma virus

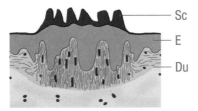

Verruca vulgaris AKA Common wart is a childhood complaint on the fingers and hands due to a viral In and may be contagious particularly on the same person spreading via the blood or contact

Venous Ulcer – breakdown of the skin due to thrombophlebitis &/or varicose veins **AKA static ulcers** *see also* **Ulcer**

vertex – top, superior point

Vesicles wrt skin fluid filled cavities in the epidermis <.5mm *see also* **Blister, Bullae Spongiosis**

Villoma AKA Papilloma warty growth with epithelial extension growth type commoner on MMs

Violacious violet colour used to describe the skin and lesions

Vitilgo chronic progressive anomaly of the skin with large hypo-pigmented patches, which may spread & are commoner on pigmented skins. It may be an AI disease or a viral In, which attacks the melanocytes – it is irreversible, on the scalp it also causes hair depigmentation – canities, leucotrichia
See also **Lentigo**

Volar relating to palms

von Reckinghausen's disease *see* **Neurofibromatosis**

Vulgar / vulgaris common plentiful, the ordinary kind

Vulva – *Lt volva = female genitals* area b/n the legs in a female that houses the external female genitalia -openings of the urethra **(U)** & vagina **(V)** and the clitoris **(C)** in the vestibule surrounded by the Labia Majora **(L maj)** and Minora **(L min)**. Hair is normally present on the Labia Majora, and around the anus **(A)** but not on the internal MM surfaces, or the opening of the anus which has much the same structure as the vermillion border of the lips.

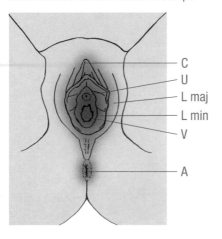

Wart = Papilloma

Seborrhoeic warts AKA Basal cell papilloma present with a flat dark warty surface & look as if stuck on the skin –appear later in life getting darker and bigger but do not become cancerous **DD BCC, melanoma, mole, solar keratoses**

Weathering – term used in hair to describe changes predominantly in the cuticle from the sun, salt, weather. Weathered hair tends to break, frizz, and split more easily and it difficult to style.

Wheal *see* **Hives & Urticaria** dermal oedema with a central pallor

White blood cells (WBC) = leucocytes general term for all blood borne cells which appear white on the blood smear includes: monocytes, lymphocytes & granulocytes *see also* **MT SKIN WOUNDED HEALING**

White head *see* **Comedo, Milium**

Whitlow In of the skin around the nail *see also* **Paronychia**

Wickham's striae *see* **Lichen**

Wood's light a UV light to see the presence of fungal spores / the depth of pigmentation in the skin *see* **Melasma**

Wrinkles On the face, 2 types **permanent** e.g. the nasolabial fold, & **dynamic** e.g. smile lines only present when the mouth is smiling. The muscles of expression attach to the subcutaneous T of the skin, so contraction causes the skin to "shorten" and form "folds", which with repetition become permanent. They run at right angles to the direction of the muscles of facial expression. Paralyzing these muscles stops skin movement.

On the body – skin must be large enough to allow for deeper movement and fat storage – with weight loss/gain & excessive movement/shaking as in exercise, excessive skin develops & folds over, forming wrinkles & skin folds, *see also* **BO-TOX, MT SKIN - Aging overview.**

xanth (ZANth)– yellow

Xanthelasma appears as yellow-orange plaques on the eyelids, from a build up of fat droplets in susceptible skin cells.

Xanthoma yellow lumps *see also* **Eruptive Xanthoma**

xero- (ZEH-roh) dry

Xerosis AKA dry skin generally referring to excessively dry skin, which cracks and scales, mainly on the UL & LL. It occurs in the older patient

Yaws AKA Thymosis, Polypapilloma tropicum, Bejel is a tropical In of the skin & bones and joints caused by the Spirochete bacterium

The bacteria appears in 3 stages – as sores on the limbs which resolve to return later in a more destructive manner and then the 3º stage when bones and cartilages are irreversibly destroyed including the nose.

Zonula Aderons (ZA) - structure connects 2 cells together and minimizes traffic b/n cells, part of the TJC. *see also* **TJC**

Zonula Occludens (ZO) - structure which connects 2 cms together and prevents any substances moving b/n the cells, part of the TJC. *see also* **TJC**

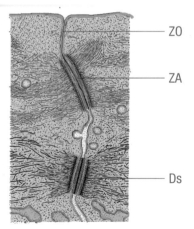

ZO

ZA

Ds

Zosteriform dermatomal rash occurring with the distribution of a N pathway

Notes

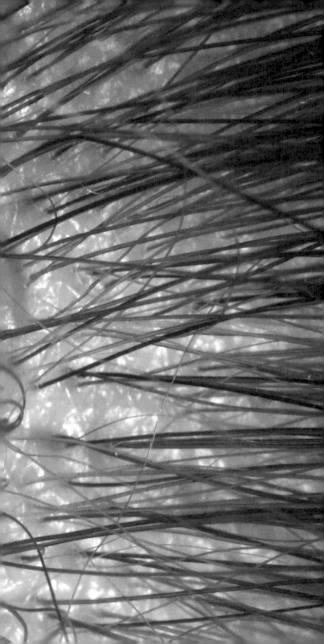

Development of the Hair Follicle –
morphogenesis

Hair morphogenesis generally is described in 8 stages pictured here. It commences in the 3rd gestational month. The first hair to develop is Lanugo hair later shed & replaced by the Vellus hair &/or Terminal hair.

Stage 0 – initial pattern layout
Induction of the overlying early epithelial cells (from the ectoderm) by the underlying dermal cells (from the mesenchyme), determines where the hair follicles will be placed, setting the pattern of the hair distribution over the body.

Stage 1– keratinocytes are induced to proliferate and the dermis develops makes way for the epithelial downgrowth

Stage 3 – mesenchymal cells induce the down growth of the epithelial cells

Stage 4 – formation of the placode

Stage 5 – commitment of cells to form subsequent specialized populations with differentiation

D = dermis
E = epithelium

1. **early epithelial cells loosely arranged on the basement membrane (BM)**
2. **specialized mesenchymal cells – part of the developing dermis – inducing change in the overlying keratinocytes**
3. **follicular papilla – hair growth inducer**
4. **epithelial downgrowth = placode**
5. **inner root sheath**
6. **sebaceous gland**
7. **"bulge"**
8. **melanin pigment**
9. **hair shaft**

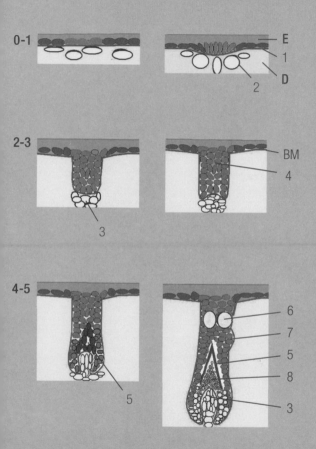

0-1
E
1
2
D

2-3
BM
4
3

4-5
6
7
5
8
3
5

Development of the Hair Follicle – morphogenesis

Stage 6 – growth accelerated by the follicular papilla with apoptosis of the intervening cells to make way for the hair shaft

Stage 7 – further differentiation if epithelial cells to form glands / bulge cells

D = dermis

E = epithelium

1 early epithelial cells loosely arranged on the basement membrane (BM)
2 specialized mesenchymal cells – part of the developing dermis – inducing change in the overlying keratinocytes
3 follicular papilla – hair growth inducer from the Dermis
4 epithelial downgrowth = placode
5 IRS
6 sebaceous gland
7 "bulge"
8 melanin pigment
9 hair shaft
10 hair bulb
11 hair follicle

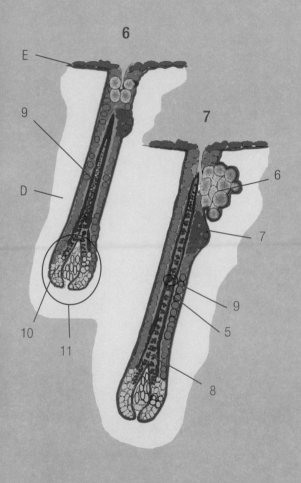

6

E

9

D

10

11

7

6

7

9

5

8

Development of the Hair Follicle – morphogenesis

Stage 8 – emergence of the fully developed hair from the follicule – coated with sebum from the sebaceous gland

D = dermis

E = epithelium

1. early epithelial cells loosely arranged on the basement membrane (BM)
2. specialized mesenchymal cells – part of the developing dermis – inducing change in the overlying keratinocytes
3. FDP
4. epithelial downgrowth = placode
5. IRS
6. sebaceous gland
7. "bulge"
8. melanin pigment
9. hair shaft

9

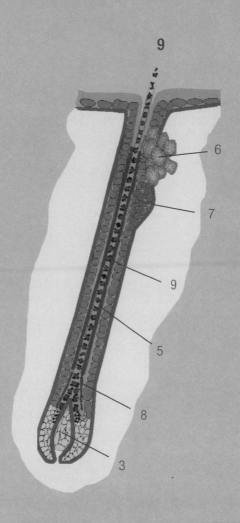

6

7

9

5

8

3

Hair Distribution – overview

Most of the body is covered with fine hair, which starts to form in the 3rd gestational month – Lanugo hair – which is shed soon after.

Glabrous areas include – lips, naval, palms, soles parts of the ear, nose & genitalia.

Lanugo hair is replaced with Vellus hair, which is shorter thinner & with a stronger cortex.

No new HFs develop after birth.

Some areas of the body develop terminal hair immediately although there may be up to 7% of vellus hair maintained in these regions throughout life, including the scalp.

Colour has a bearing on the amount of hair on the head & body – with the scalp representing 2% of the total body hair. Generally blondes have the most hair follicles / skin area, but this may vary with ethnic origin.

Intermediate hair is a transitional stage hair type seen in the conversion of vellus to terminal hair.

Androgenic transformation of vellus hairs takes place at puberty & may continue slowly into the 30s. In the female after menopause the female pattern may vary to include some features of the male pattern including scalp hair loss.

Short terminal hairs appear on the limbs, chest, back & face as well as around the axilla & genitals, with puberty, and this conversion can continue to increase for several years after.

Changes at puberty

Changes continuing after puberty into 30s

Changes with the menopause

Changes with age > 60

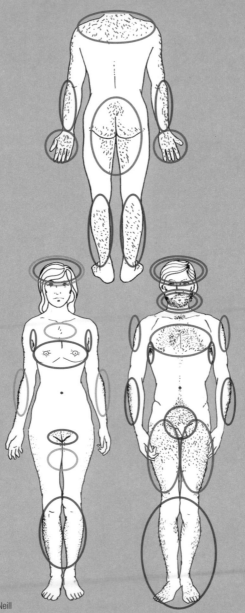

© A. L. Neill

Hair Growth Cycle – overview

Hair growth cycle – commences after the formation of the hair follicle (HF) "in utero, "Lanugo hair.

This HF ⬇ by 30% (Catagen) rests (Telogen) & is shed – with the new HF formed which commences the first of its life cycles, repeated until the final death of the hair, either vellus or terminal.

CATAGEN 1– Pilo-sebaceous unit = mini-organ Hair follicle (HF) suicide 1:1000 hairs

Melanogenesis ceases & melanocytes die, but the keratinocytes of the hair matrix (HM) continue to grow slowly de-pigmented. Then the keratinocytes also die in a group creating a gap b/n the HS & the follicular dermal papilla (FDP). As the HM dies it drags up the FDP to the level of the bulge (B).

The HF is now 30% of its size.

TELOGEN 2- Resting stage 1:10 hairs

The hair unit seems inactive but new specialized cells are developing: root sheaths, melanocytes & hair matrix epithelium (HM). The new HF starts to move downwards from B.

EXOGEN 3 active extrusion of old HF 100-200 hairs daily are shed

Active shedding of the old HF commences before the tip of the new HS has reached it. This is an active hair shedding event, which overlaps with Anagen.

ANAGEN 4 – active hair shaft growth 8 :10 hairs

Great ⬆ keratinocyte proliferation directed by the new FDP. Formation of a new HS composed of pressed dead cells arranged as: the cuticle, cortex & medulla.

D = dermis E = epithelium

_____ movement of the HF _____ movement of the HS

1 arrector pili muscle
2 sebaceous gland
3 "bulge"
4 outer root sheath
5 inner root sheath
6 HS
7 melanin granules / pigment

8 follicular dermal papilla (FDP)
9 hair matrix – keratinocytes associated with the FDP
10 regressing keratinocyte bridge b/n old & new FDP
11 de-pigmented terminal HS
12 club hair

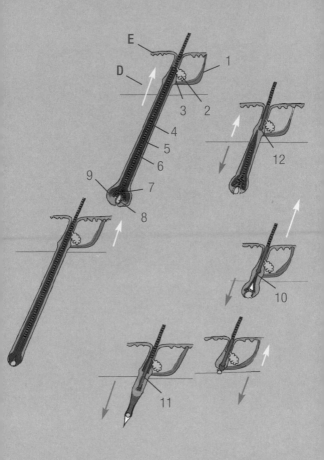

Scalp Hair Loss - miniaturization

Male scalp hair loss is generally due to androgenic alopecia - a form of HAIR THINNING.

The terminal scalp hairs change to fine less pigmented vellus hair
   1 moving up from the subcutaneous T to the upper dermis.
   2 reducing in diameter from 60 μm to < 20μm
   3 shortening the anagen & cycling progressively quicker & quicker. until disappearing altogether.
   4 losing pigment & medulla with reduced follicle size

This is generally slow and not accompanied by obvious hair shedding – i.e. hair found in brushes or on pillows etc. White hair is less susceptible than brown hair & so the hair seems lighter in the thinning areas.

The pattern generally starts from the crown but also there is loss of the frontal hairline – moving in sequence from 1-7 with preservation of hair in area 7 which overlies large muscle mass on the scalp.

Scalp Hair Loss - effluvium

Females are generally more susceptible to this form of hair loss which is defined as the active shedding of hair in the telogen phase – exogen. It lasts 3 – 6mnths time for the new anagen hair to re-emerge. It's triggered by: Hormones – as in pregnancy & menopause, physiological & psychological stresses & vitamin deficiencies.

Large amounts of hair are detected falling out or being released with minor pulling. It does not usually produce bald areas but a diffuse thinning. When hair is pulled, if there is >25% in Telogen it denotes effluvian (normal is b/n 5-15%). It is usually reversible with recovery from the stressor, or removal of the trigger, unless it is the beginning of female pattern baldness

Female pattern baldness differs from the male - in that there is a diffuse loss - with frontal hairline sparing. Often one of the first signs is a widening part line – followed by thinner hair at the vertex but w/o an obvious "bald spot."

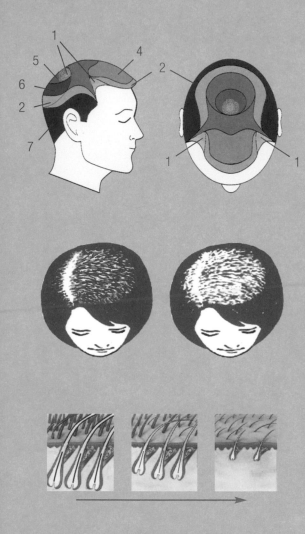

HAIR BONDS

The Hydrogen Bond
Responsible for 35% of the HS's strength & its elasticity.
Located b/n the alpha helix coils.

The Salt Bond
Responsible for 35% of the HS's strength.
Ionic bond b/n 2 amino acids.

The Cystine Bond – disulphide bond
Covalent links b/n 2 amino acids – generally cystine.
Cysteine-SH + HS-Cysteine <—> Cysteine-S-S-Cysteine = CYSTINE + H_2

The number and site of the sulphur bonds determines the "curl" of the hair. Breakage and reformation of the sulphur bonds are used in permanent waving and straightening procedures.
They are spaced along the HS in straight hair and more and more asymmetrically in curlier and curlier hair

The Sugar Bond
Responsible for the moisture content of the hair.
A bond b/n an acid and alkaline in the hair.

HAIR ELASTICITY

Dry Hair
A Good hair can be stretched up to 45% reversibly
C Poor hair has very little elasticity – breaks easily and does not regain its shape
B Most hair falls in b/n particularly if it has been treated

Wet Hair
Has more elasticity up to 60% – but is more fragile

1	normal length	3	wet hair
2	stretched hair	4	stretched wet hair

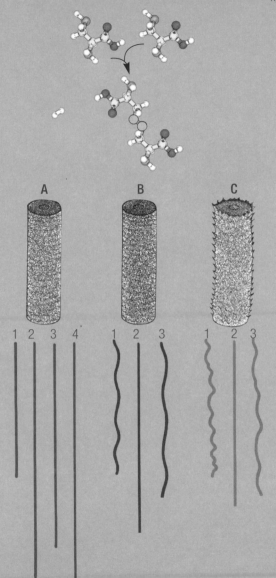

Hair Greying / Hair Tinting

Hair has its own natural colour, derived from the melanin granules injected into the cortex by the melanocytes of the hair matrix in the bulb. **EUMELANIN** is the commoner coming in 2 types the brown & black forms. **PHEOMELANIN** is the other form responsible for pink to red shades in the hair & skin. These remain in the amorphous protein of the cortex held there by the cuticle which itself is transparent.

Melanin is derived from tyrosine. It is: granular, water insoluble, smaller than haeme breakdown products (.8µm), a semi-conductor, a strong metal binding ligand, and UV light & sound absorber.

Eumelanin
(part of)

Pheomelanin (part of)

Hair in poor condition – i.e. porous cuticle lose their melanin / colour with washing.

Canities – greying hair occurs when the melanocytes cease producing granules for the HS for an extended period and the first sign of impending catogen is the cessation of melanin in the HS.

Canities normally occurring around middle-age can be accelerated by anxiety & hereditary factors. It is generally irreversible but not linked with thinning or shedding, although these factors may independently cause these events. Because of the increased spaces in the cotex - greying hair is easier to tint.

In order to permanently re-colour / tint the hair – the dye must penetrate the cuticle and lodge in the cortex. Covering the cuticle with dye will wear off and wash off immediately.

1 permanent dye
2 semi-permanent dye
3 medulla
4 melanin granules
5 HS in good condition – with intact cuticle
6 HS in poor condition – cuticle vulnerable –
   dyes come in and go out

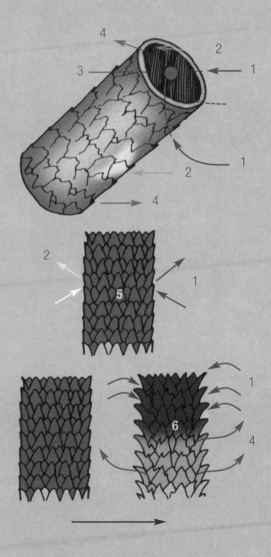

Hair Structure – terminal hair

Angle = the angle of the hair follicle determines the way it grows, the straighter the angle the straighter the hair – generally the curlier hairs grow out increasingly acute angles

Hair bulb (HB) = the portion of living hair attached to the lowest part of the follicle = the epidermal matrix just above the FDP

Hair bulge = extension of the ORS, site of muscle attachment

Hair follicle (HF) = a tube-shaped indentation from the epidermis from the base of the dermal papilla & extending deep into the dermis - length varies.

Hair matrix (HM) = epidermal matrix = keratinocytes directly above the FDP (papilla) - these actively dividing cells form the HS & have embedded in them melanocytes which inject melanin pigment into the cortex of the hair

Hair root (HR) = the part of the hair enclosed entirely w/n the follicle – epithelial origin

Hair shaft (HS) = the dead part of the unit – the hair just above the bulb to the visible hair

Papilla = follicle dermal papilla (FDP) = the dermal cell origin which induces the growth and formation of the hair by the surrounding keratinocytes – this is the only vascularised area of the hair.

Sebaceous gland = gland attached to the hair shaft secreting sebum – generally located on the side of the arrector pili muscle & angle of the hair growth. It contains up to 8 sacs with a common neck – it lies on a BM as do all epithelial structures.

1 Sc
2 E
3 Du
4 arrector pili muscle, changes the Angle of the HF, pulls the skin and causes *goosebumps*
5 sebaceous gland
6 "bulge"
7 fibrocollagenous follicle sheath – modified BM
8 melanin granules/pigment
9 hair matrix – keratinocytes
   associated with the FDP
10 FDP / hair follicle
11 melanocytes
12 IRS, ORS
13 glassy membrane continuous with the BM
14 HS consists of 3 parts -
14m medulla
14c cortex
14cu cuticle
15 pore infundibulum for hair emergance

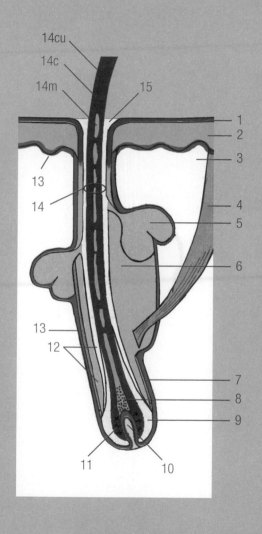

14cu

14c

14m

15

1

2

3

13

14

4

5

6

13

12

7

8

9

11

10

Hair Structure - regions Terminal Hair in Anagen

The hair unit = pilosebaceous unit is a mini- organ. It has many site specific regions where considerable differentiation & cyclical processes take place.

1 SCorneum (Sc)
2 Epithelium (E)
3 upper dermis / papillary dermis (Du)
4 arrector pili muscle
5 eccrine sweat gland sebaceous gland
6 sebaceous gland
7 dermal BVs & N
8 bulge – extension of the ORS
9 HS
10 root sheaths o = outer (ORS) i = inner (IRS)
11 glassy membrane – separating E & mesenchymal sections continuous with the BM
12 mesenchymal sheath – containing copious free N endings-& BVs
13 hair bulb = IRS + matrix keratinocytes
14 follicle dermal papilla (FDP)

A permanent section of HF from surface to insertion of arrector pili muscle
Ai infundibulum – surface to the insertion of the sebaceous gland
Aia acroinfundibulum – upper part of the infundibulum – includes opening on the surface limit of the Sc + Sg layers
Aii infrainfundibulum – loss of distinct E layers – narrowing of the HS
Ais isthmus region b/n the gland & the bulge
 narrowed HS; end of the IRS;
 site of hardening keratins in the ORS determining the X sectional shape of the hair
B deep cyclical section –in anagen it is in the subcutaneous fat moves up to the dermis in catogen
Bb bulbar region
Bs suprabulbar region

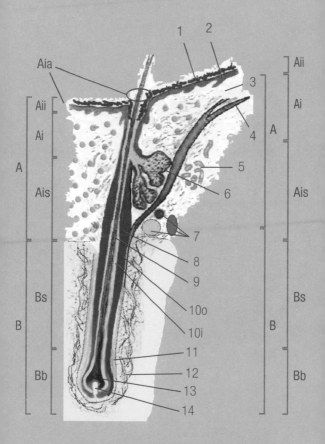

Aia

Aii
Ai
A
Ais

B
Bs

Bb

1   2

3
4

5
6

7
8
9

10o
10i

11
12
13
14

Aii
Ai
A
Ais

B
Bs

Bb

Hair follicle - Blood Supply

The HF is derived both from the dermis and epidermis. Like the epidermis the HF has no direct BVs, but is supplied from BVs in the dermis, the hair bulb (HB) is supplied by the follicular dermal papilla (FDP) and along the shaft via diffusion from the nearby dermal T, at all times separated by the BM or the glassy membrane.

1. E
2. BM / glassy membrane - modified BM along the HS
3. dermal papilla
4. vascular plexus
   d = deep s = superficial
5. reticular dermis
6. sebaceous gland
7. FDP
8. subcutaneous fatty tissue
9. HB - note BVs surround the bulb
10. junctional zone & pore infundibulum - epidermis continues down the HS and contains progenitor cells which help with skin maintenance and repair

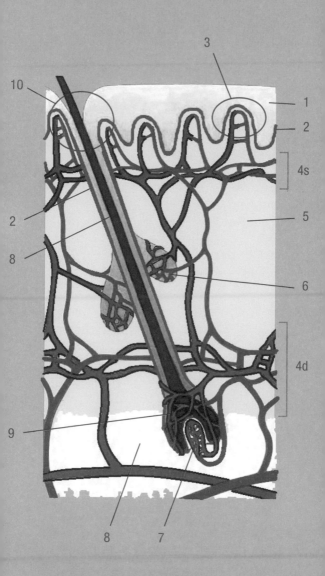

Hair Bulb Microstructure – terminal hair

Longitudinal / cross section

The hair is an epidermal structure but it is supported by the dermis.

The BS comes via the papilla – a dermal structure. There is no direct BS to the hair

The hyaline layer protects & supports the HS, directing its growth / expansion & isolating it from the dermis. The internal & external root shafts do not progress past the skin surface, only the HS structures which consist of dead keratinocytes and melanin pigments.

- 0 **Hyaline layer – acellular layer b/n the Hair & supportive surrounding tissue AKA glassy membrane (extension of the BM)**
- 1 **outer dermal layer – dermis around the Hair**
- 2 **ORS containing stem cells**
- 3 **Henle's layer**
- 4 **Huxleys layer**

3 + 4 = IRS

HAIR SHAFT

- 5 **cuticle**
- 6 **cortex**
- 7 **medulla**

HAIR BULB

- 8 **focal dermal papilla (FDP)**
- 9 **BVs supplying the papilla**
- 10 **hair follicle surrounding the dermal papilla**

CELL TYPES

- 11 **keratinocyte populations**
- 12 **melanocytes**
- 13 **cell debris**
- 14 **melanin pigments**
- 15 **fibroblasts**

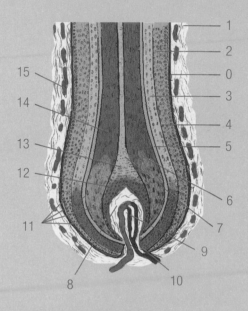

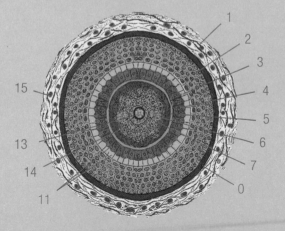

Hair Cortex & Medulla

The Cortex of the hair is responsible for its texture, of which there are 3 main types.

A FINE ~.04 mm diameter
B MEDIUM ~.08 mm diameter
C COARSE ~.12mm diameter

Cells are long cylinders 50 -100µm X 3-6 µm with interdigitating teeth to join them, in an amorphous protein gel with high sulphur containing protein content.

The Medulla is a tube filled with air & contains the protein trichohyaline.

It acts as an excretory tool – containing debris of the hair formation – & poisons from the body AT THE TIME are actively extruded into this area, where they remain. Hence it becomes a window of activity of that time, and a great forensic tool.

It is hydrophilic and will absorb and keep moisture if it penetrates through the cuticle. This swelling may distort the entire shape of the HS.

D DOUBLE MEDULLAE see often in Asian hair

E SINGLE REGULAR MEDULLA common in terminal & short medium or coarse scalp hair

F BROKEN MEDULLA common in treated hair (also swollen)

G ABSENT MEDULLA – common in vellus hair or fine scalp hair

1 cuticle
2 cortex
3 medulla

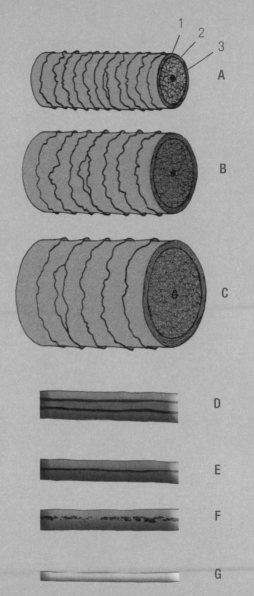

Hair Structure – cuticle

The cuticle of the Hair shaft (HS) is transparent, and it acts to protect the inner structures and pigments, in the cortex. It consists of a series of overlapping "roof tiles" or "shingles" which are plates of keratinocytes pointing away from the root at ~ 5^0 bound to each other via fatty acids and covalent bonds.

It contains b/n 7-10 layers & is thickest in straight, short, terminal hairs.

It may appear shiny as it reflects light & coloured as it transmits the pigments in the cortex. These properties are most enhanced in scalp hair.

The porosity of the HS depends upon how tightly these plates are adherent.

Porosity is the ability of the HS to absorb moisture irrespective of its texture.

With age – and length from the surface these tiles become looser & looser and this change is irreversible.

Weathering is the term used for this change.

Weathering ⬆ with hair length, exposure to sun and water particularly salt water; with friction caused by brushing particularly with metal brushes, colouring & treatments which alter the curl or shape of the HS.

⬆ weathering = ⬆ porosity = ⬇ elasticity of the hair =
⬆ ability to absorb moisture = ⬇ shine on the hair

A = poor porosity – closed cuticle scales - resistant to treatment, hard to tint

B = medium porosity – normal hair, most hair responds to colouring treatment

C = good porosity – long hair – very good take up of tint

D = extreme porosity – fragile hair likely to break - takes up tints well but also loses them because of poor cuticle integrity

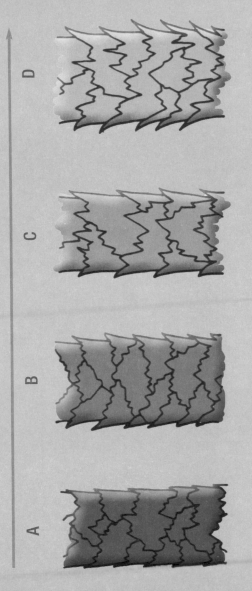

A B C D

Hair Structure – cuticle layers

The cuticle of the Hair shaft (HS) is transparent, and it acts to protect the inner structures and pigments, in the cortex. It consists of a series of overlapping "roof tiles" or "shingles" which are plates of keratinocytes pointing away from the root at ~ 5° bound to each other via lipids consisting of fatty acids (palmitic, stearic, & oleic) and wax esters. The bonds b/n these substances are degraded by UV light.

Size of the cuticle 50 X 0.5 micrometers.

Initially it contains b/n 7-10 layers but on long hairs may be only 2-3 layers.

These scales point downwards so that it is possible to stroke hair one way w/o resistance but not the other, which is why straight hair generally has stronger thicker cuticles.

Cross section of the hair layers include :

CUTICLE LAYERS (Cu)

1 **external surface**

2 **epicuticle = semi-permeable membrane of the HS**

3 **A layer = sulphur rich proteins = cystine makes up 30%**

4 **exocuticle = suphur proteins make up 15% - gives mechanical stability**

5 **endocuticle = absorb water, hydrophilic causes the cuticle to swell and loose its surface plates**

OTHER

6 **cell membrane = lipid bipolar layer strongly adherent joining the cuticle and cortex**

7 **cortex = long keratin shafts impregnated with melanin pigments**

8 **medulla (may be absent – in fine and vellus hair) – thin hollow section**

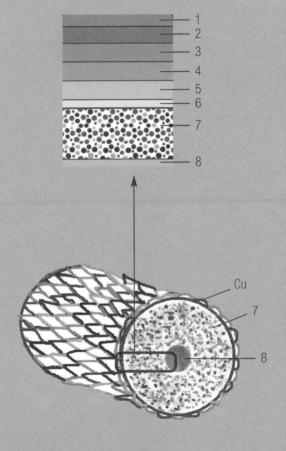

Hair Shaft (HS)

The HS is composed of dead keratinocytes.

The Stratum germinativum is the anlagen of this structure – forming its 3 components.

1 The cuticle composed of: curved, flattened, overlapping, adherent, transparent corneocytes – (keratinocytes devoid of any intracellular structures and filled with keratin).

2 The cortex composed of: long, keratin fibrils impregnated with melanin pigments.

3 The medulla composed of: air & the protein – trichohyalin.

4 pigment – derived from melanin – high molecular – water insoluble (note this is the same pigment basis of the skin only in the skin it remains intracellular)

> **phaeomelanin** = red & yellow pigments
> **eumelanin** = brown & black pigments

5 exposed cortex – after the loss of a cuticle – due to weathering or UV destruction etc.

Note when the cortex is exposed, the HS is very vulnerable to damage

– the cortex may lose filaments &/or pigment

– the medulla may swell as it is hydrophilic causing further cuticle lift off and starting a vicious cycle of HS splitting. breakage & loss.

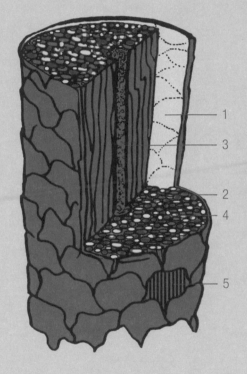

1

3

2

4

5

Hair Shaft Microstructure

Hair is 88% protein derived from keratin.

Keratin is composed of polypeptide chains arranged in an "alpha helix" **(1)**.

These are then twisted together to form a protofibril **(2)**. The 1st actual "hairfibre"

9 protofibrils then are bound in a circle and these circles **(3)** then are bound around each other to form a "microfibril" **(4)**.

Microfibrils are embedded in an amorphous protein matrix of high sulphur content **(5)**.

100s of microfibrils are cemented into an irregular fibrous bundle called a "macrofibril" **(6)** Many of these macrofibrils are formed inside the keratinocyte **(7)** at the base of the HS, which then is elongated, dehydrated and it dies. This is pushed up the HS, along with its nuclear remnants **(8)** along with the remains of its cytoplasm complex **(9)**. This whole structure forms the cortex along with melanin pigments inserted from the melanocytes at the hair base.

Packed dead cells surround these structures & form the cuticle **(10)**

In the centre of these structures lies the medulla. This is a canal which is actually a part of the hair & body's excretory system. It concentrates the debris of the forming HS & acts as a repository for other debris such as: drug metabolites, heavy metals, synthetics & medications.

1 **alpha helix**

2 **protofibril**

3 **circle**

4 **microfibril**

5 **protein matrix**

6 **macrofibril**

7 **dehyrated keratinocyte**

8 **nuclear remnant**

9 **cell membrane**

10 **cuticle**

    10p epicuticle

    10A layer which determines the extent of the wave of the hair

    10n endocuticle

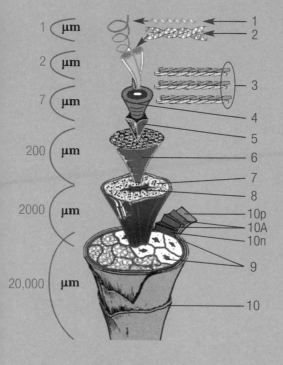

1 μm   1
2 μm   2
7 μm   3
     4
     5
200 μm   6
     7
     8
2000 μm   10p
     10A
     10n
     9
20,000 μm   10

Hair Types

There are 2 main types of hair. **VELLUS & TERMINAL**

Other types –

Intermediate – transitional hair when converting from vellus to terminal hair & visa versa as in the miniaturization process – male balding.

Lanugo – primitive hair developing in utero – 3rd gestational month, may re-emerge in severe disease states particularly of malnutrition.

Under the correct conditions these types are all interchangeable. However conversion of vellus to short terminal hairs is generally not reversible, on the body.

The FDP determines the length and type of hair growth – its cycle and age. The epithelial cells are influenced but do not determine the hair type they will become.

	lanugo	vellus	terminal
percentage of total HFs	100 until birth	95	5 – (2 scalp hair)
HS diameter	+++	+	++++ - ++++++
HS morphology	globular/fine	curved	highly variable
HS Xsection	irregular	circular	flat, elliptical, oval, circular
HS length	2 - 6cm	2 - 3cm	1- 60cm
HB location	upper dermis	dermis	subcutaneous T
FDP	10-50 cells	10-30 cells	300-400 cells
Hair BS	local diffusion	diffusion from surrounding T	BVs to the FDP
perifollicular structures	–	2 - 6	0
Hyaline layer b/n hair & CT support		+++	+
Pigmentation	0 - 1	0 - 2	0 - 6
Cuticle layers	1 - 2	2 - 4	4 - 10
Cuticle damage	–	+	⬆ with hair length, shape & treatments
Medulla	0	0 - 1	1 - 2
Growth phase (Anagen)	weeks	months	weeks – 10 years
Growth type	synchronized	mosaic	mosaic – but constant for each hair unless stressed
Growth rate	–	.2mm/day	.2-1mm /day
Resting phase (Telogen)	–	weeks - months	weeks
Androgen sensitivity	nil	2	2-4
Age changes	nil	few	extensive – pigment changes, canities, loss ⬆, texture changes, density changes ⬆ or ⬇ regionally related, Anagen ⬇, Telogen ⬆
Sensitivity to external conditions	only in extreme conditions	few	extensive – hair may shed / change pigment / thin / medullary changes
Sebaceous glands	–	1 - 2 / HF	1 - 6 / HF
Apocrine glands	–	–	0 - 4 / HF
Arrector pili muscle	–	1/ HF	0
Nerve endings		extensive & specialized	minimal
Immune status		protected	protected

© A. L. Neill

Hair Regional Types – overview

There are 2 basic hair types vellus & terminal – however there are also regional changes of HFs.

Terminal hair may be short :– eyelash, eyebrow, nasal or ear or long:- scalp or beard. The texture may be coarse, medium or fine depending upon the diameter of the shaft.

It is to be noted that "donor site "dominates so that if the hair is transplanted it generally maintains its original regional type and this is why scalp hair transplants are possible.

1– Pubic / Axillary hairs Short, medium terminal hairs convert from vellus hairs with ⬆androgen levels at puberty. They are associated with apocrine sweat glands as well as eccrine glands. Anagen is a matter of months.

2- Eyelash hairs Short coarse curved terminal hairs found around the eye have minimal glands & are replaced every 2-3 months.

3 – Nasal / Ear canal hairs Short coarse terminal hairs become larger / longer ⬆androgens. They have a close association with mucosal glands & sebaceous glands.

4 – Vellus hairs Fine thin hairs are found over most of the body, >96%. They are in Du, papillae < 2cm, ⬇pigmentation, no medulla, ⬇ cuticle but can be transformed into terminal hairs with ⬆ androgen influence.

5 – Scalp / Beard hairs Long terminal hairs make up 2% of the body's total hairs. ⬆pigmented, ⬆cuticles 7-10 layers. The Beard hairs are the fastest growing up to 1mm/day, but Scalp hairs have the longest Anagen up to 10 years, which determines their maximal length.

6- Glabrous areas Areas on the body which do not grow hair – vermilion zone of the lips, palms, soles behind the ears

Hair does not grow on the palms & soles as the SCorneum layer is so thick & the dermal papillae so shallow and distorted that hair induction cannot take place.

A = apocrine glands   D = dermis,   Du = upper dermis,
Dp = dermal papilla   E = epithelium   FDP = follicular dermal papilla,
G = sebaceous gland,   H = hair shaft   M = mucus glands
s = sweat glands   Sc = Stratum corneum   Su subcutaneous fat

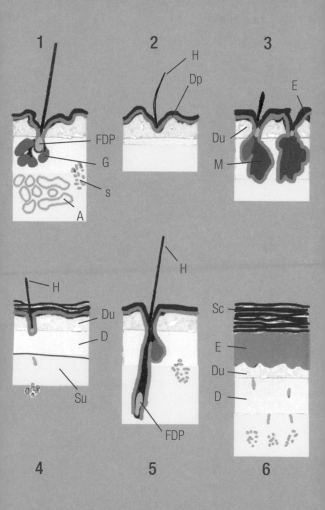

1

FDP

G

s

A

2

H

Dp

3

E

Du

M

4

H

Du

D

Su

5

H

FDP

6

Sc

E

Du

D

Scalp Hair types –

	STRAIGHT			WAVY		
Distribution	Caucasian	Mixed	Asian	Mixed	Mixed	Mixed
type	1a	1b	1c	2a	2b	2c
texture	fine/thin	medium	coarse	fine/thin	medium	coarse
shaft crossection						
shaft line						
rate of growth	.7mm/day +++	.7mm/day +++	.7mm/day ++	0-.7mm/day ++	0-.7mm/day ++	0-.7mm/day ++
oilyness	++++	+++	+	++	++	+
strength	+++	+++	+++	++	++	++
ability to "style"	++++	+++	+	++++	+++	++
tendency to frizz (cuticle fragility)	+	+	+	+	+	+
elasticity	+++	++	+	+++	++	+
colour						
special features	even disulphide bonds	even disulphide bonds	even disulphide bonds			

© A. L. Neill

	CURLY		KINKY	
Distribution	Caucasian	Mixed	Asian	Mixed
type	3a	3b	4a	4b
texture	loose curls	tight curls	soft	wiry
shaft crossection				
shaft line				
rate of growth	0-.7mm/day +	0-.7mm/day +	<.4mm/day	<.3mm/day
oilyness	++	++	+	+
strength	++	++	+	+
ability to "style"	++	+	+	+
tendency to frizz (cuticle fragility)	+++	+++++	++++++	++++++
elasticity	++	+	+	+
colour				
special features			may felt absent medulla	may felt absent medulla

Notes

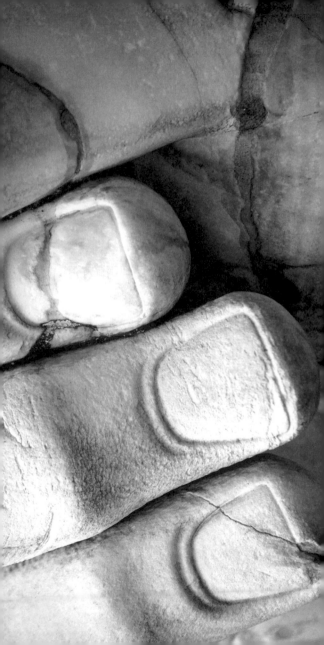

Nail Anatomy

The nail like hair is composed of keratin and "dead" except at the root.

The rate of growth depends upon the length of the distal phalange hence – the index finger is the fastest growing and the little toe the slowest. Rate of growth is b/n 1-3mm/mnth, faster in the summer and in good nutrition.

1   body of the nail = nail plate

2   nail moon = lunula

3c cuticle = eponychium

3e free edge of the cuticle = perionyx

4   nail sinus

5   nail root = germinal matrix = onychostroma

6   E

7   Du

8   subcutaneous T / fat

9   distal phalange

10 quick = hyponychium

11 nail bed

12 free edge of the nail = margo liber

13 joint capsule & surrounding ligaments

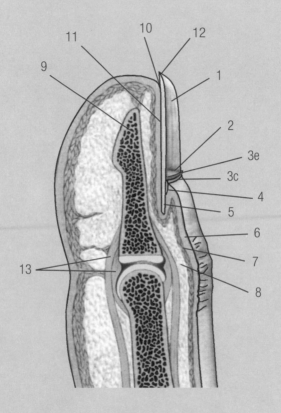

Nail Anatomy – dorsal surface

The nail's function is to protect the finger-tip, extend the precision grip to the level of the free nail edge, and increase the accuracy of the precision – and to act as a counter weight in grips using the fingertips. Nails are not claws, although related to them, they are better designed for balance and enhancing specialized grips than aggression.

1   free edge of the nail = margo liber = distal edge of nail plate

2   quick = hyponychium

3   body of the nail = nail plate

4   onychodermal band = b/n the nail bed and the quick

5   nail root = germinal matrix = onychostroma under the proximal nail fold

6   matrix crests = nail grooves

7   cuticle = eponychium & free edge of the cuticle = perionyx

8   nail sinus

9   lunula = visible portion of the nail matrix

10 lateral nail fold

11 proximal nail fold

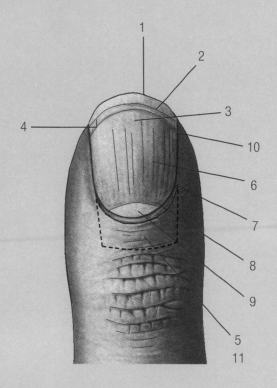

Nail Anatomy – Growth patterns HP

The finger & toe nails are modified claws & hooves respectively.

The NP in the human is flatter – thinner and more porous, than the claw. Replacement time for the finger nail is b/n 3-6 mnths & toenail up to 2X as long.

The NM is responsible for the NP, cuticle & skin folds around it.

1 epidermis = Sc + BM
2 dermis
3 proximal nail fold
4 eponychium
5 cuticle + its free edge = perionyx
6 nail plate =unguis
7 onychodermal junction
8 sole plate = subunguis
9 free nail edge = margo liber
10 quick = hyponychium
11 finger tip
12 finger pulp – dermis – site of the glomus bodies – av shunts of the fingers
13 nail bed (NB)
14 nail matrix (NM) – root of the nail

The thicker the NM the thicker the NP; distal onychocytes grow up and around to form the surface of the NP as they flatten, lose their nuclei and form clear transparent plates with intervening fibres and protein matrix, similar to the hair shaft. Persistence of the nuclei will result in softer spongier white nails – parakeratosis.

1 NM onychocytes
2 NM
3 NP
4 free edge of the NP
5 hyponychium
6 NB

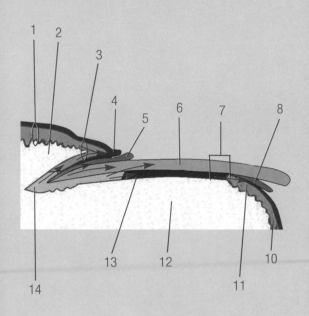

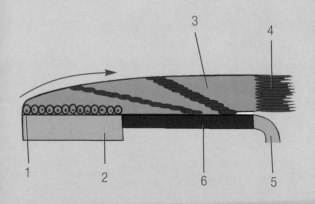

Nail Growth Rates

Fingernails take b/n 3-6 mnths to replace & toenails at least 2X longer. Thicker NP are due to thicker NM – the surface layers coming from the deepest cells.

Faster growth	Slower growth
Deeper NM	Shallow NM
Youth	Aging
♂ Pregnancy Daytime	♀ Lactation Night
⬆temp, summer; Minor trauma (piano, typing, nail biting)	⬇temp, winter Immobilization of digit
⬆BS (AV shunt) Dominant hand, 3rd finger	⬇BS, poor circulation diseases, DM
Premenses Psoriasis Regeneration after loss	Inflammation chronic or acute, Chronic diseases, malnutrition, Paralysis, Peripheral neuropathy Brittle nail syndrome, Yellow nail syn; Lichen planus
Meds Ca, Vit D, benoxaprofen, levodopa, biotin, cysteine, retinoids, antifungals	**Meds**, gold, gold, lithium, sulfonamides, heparin

Abnormal Direction

Hook Nail - bowing of NB due to lack of support from short bony phalanx

Mal-alignment of NP - common. Congenital: big toe; lat deviation of long axis of nail growth relative to distal phalanx. Other causes: trauma

Onychocryptosis - ingrown nails; distal ingrowing - big toe esp at birth

Onychauxis - hypertrophied nails 2° to trauma & pressure

Onychophosis – hyperkeratosis on the subunguis ± NF, 1st or 5th toes; trauma

1	NP	3	NB
2	NM	4	onychokeratinization plane

© A. L. Neill

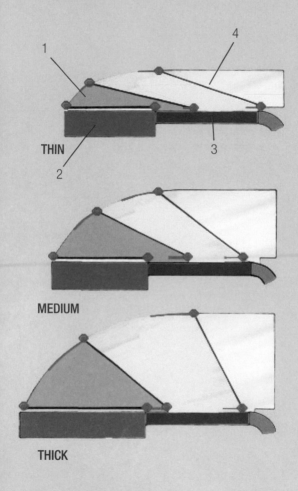

1

4

2

THIN

3

MEDIUM

THICK

Nail Plate Growth

The NP grows over the NB – which is composed of grooved epithelial cells, lying on a tightly fixed dermis. The epithelial cells slide along with the NP providing nourishment via the highly vascular dermis underneath – it does not have BVs of its own.

It does not contribute to the NP cells.*

1 **NP top layer – water moves through the plate and is evaporated from this surface**
2 **NP – filled with gaps & channels allows passage of substances – both ways – so lifting the layers in constant water immersion**
3 **NB – epidermal layers – grooved to fit into the NP grooves**
4 **dermis**
5 **BM**
6 **CT anchors from the dermis to the bone – stopping its movement with nail growth**

* `although this is disputed particularly in cases of parakeratosis where some cells sloughed off may be replaced by the NB

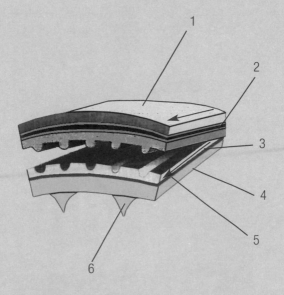

Abnormal Nail Plate Attachment

Anonychia (Absence of the nail) absence of all or part of ≥ 1 nail

I Onychogryphosis (Nail thickening) – yellow nails
Causes: eczema, onychomycosis, psoriasis, trauma
In toenails
Causes: acute trauma, chronic P from footwear, familial

II Onycholysis: (nail lifting ± pitting)
Defn: distal +/or lat separation of the NP from the tip of the NB subungual space gathers dirt / keratin debris; greyish-white colour = air under the nail disrupting the onychodermal band. Causes:
primary

1	trauma	3	Candida pseudomonas In
2	manicure	4	hereditary / familial

Causes: secondary

1	dermatoses	3	work related – partic working with water
2	medical conditions: ⬇periph circ, ▽thyroid function, hyperhidrosis	4	drugs / medication

III Onychomadesis: (nail shedding)
Defn: Complete loss of NP due to proximal nail separation which extends distally; a progression of profound Beau's lines
Causes:

1 local & generalized dermatoses
2 trauma;
3 iatrogenic: overdoses of retinoids; cloxacillin

Onychomycosis: (fungal In of nails) will cause subungual hyperkeratosis and so lifting of the nail from its bed

IV Pterygium: (destruction of the NM)
Defn: Advance of skin over the NP because of NM destruction – scar T develops and the skin grows forward but it is not a cuticle & cannot be pushed back, as there is no nail beneath
Causes:

1	trauma including toxins (Formaldehyde) from manicures	3	purulent In
		4	neuropathic damage
2	digital ischaemia	5	leprosy
		6	Raynaud's

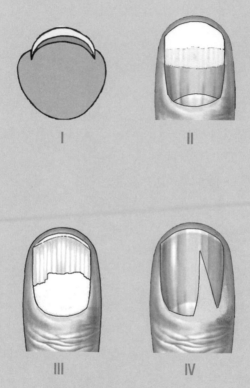

I

II

III

IV

Abnormal Nail Shape

Clubbing (Nail bending over the finger tip ⬆ nail longitudinal curvature and the finger pulp of the tip) associated with ⬆ central cyanosis & lung carcinoma

Pseudoclubbing: shortening of fingernail – after chemical exposure subungual tumor, pseudocyst,or osteoid osteoma;

Thyroid acropachy: thickening of soft Ts of hands + feet; periosteal new bone formation occurs in hands + feet rather than long bones

Shell-nail syndrome: atrophy of bone & NB; + yellow nails + clubbing

Koilonychia (spoon shaped) - due to thin NP

concave dorsal nail; esp thumb or great toe

physiological in infants resolves spontaneously

1st 3 fingernails occupational origin e.g. mechanics; hairdressers; thinning of the NP due to work solutions

trichothyodystrophy – abnormalities in the hair / from the B / thyroid 2º to Ins Psoriasis & fungi cause subungual hyperkeratosis which push up nail

Pincer / Trumpet nails (claw shaped) v painful due to trauma of ill-fitting shoes usually, familial

Macronychia (Local gigantism; racket thumb) –large nail on 1 or more digits

local giantism

premature closure of the epiphyseal line

Micronychia (small nail) generally due to an underlying bone abnormality

A - normal
B - koilonychia
C - transverse lines = Beau's lines
D - clubbing
E - pincer

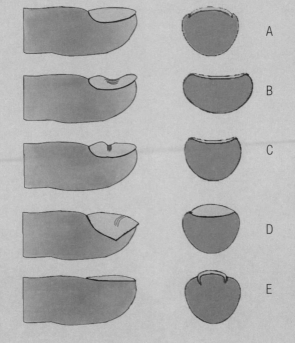

A

B

C

D

E

Abnormal Nail Surface

Grooves

I **Onychorrhexis** supf grooves that lead to distal splitting
Longitudinal grooves
Habitual tic - due to pushing back cuticle
Canal (single wide groove) - myxoid cyst Trauma, retinoids, familial
Physiological furrows (= **ridge**) exacerbated old ages

II Transverse grooves & Beau's lines
Endogenous: arcuate margin matches **lunula** congenital
Exogenous: margin matches **prox. NF**
isolated digits – trauma (e.g. manicure)
generalized digits – systemic illnesses, ⬇nutrition
measure position of grooves, to date previous illness
recurrent diseases will produce recurrent grooves

III Onychia Punctata = Pitting - foci of parakeratoses generalized -
associated with: Psoriasis, Reiter's, AA;
single, large, full-thickness pit = **elkonyxis** - seen in psoriasis.
Reiters, trauma
irregular with Xridging + discolouration - eczema, chronic paronychia,
fungal Ins

IV Trachyonychia – AKA 2° nail dystrophy = rough nails /
sandpaper - due to generalized small pitting similar to the above
causes and associations

V Onychoschizia: Lamellar dystrophy / transverse splitting into
layers at or near free edge / with discolouration due to debris
accumulation

Brittle nails together with **onychoschizia** - & assoc with water
immersion – alkaline in partic

Beading & ridging – with rheumatoid arthritis & age

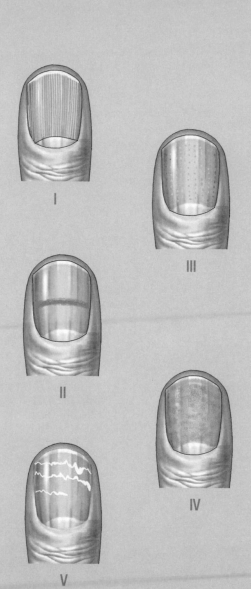

I

III

II

IV

V

Abnormal Nail Colour – brown - black

I   Melanonychia (Dark nails due to melanin deposition)

Causes – melanocyte proliferation – due to: racial variants, skin hyperpigmentation, melanoma, pigmented naevi in the NB

II   Addison's disease

III Drugs (chemo & antipsychotic) e.g. tetracycline

IV   Hyperkeratosis beneath the nail with debris = subungual hyperkeratosis

V   Infections
pseudomonas - also produce green nails

VI   Metabolic
jaundice

VII Metal deposits
pigment from metals extruded into the NP - bands are often longitudinal e.g. gold

VIII Trauma

IX   Deficiencies
Vitamin B12 defic

X   Exogenous pigment = external staining on the upper surface: colour only on the surface - with time will show a proximal band of unstained nail = quitter's nail e.g. nicotine nails

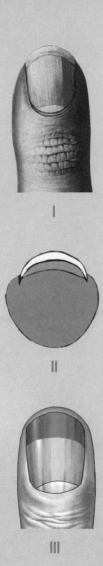

I

II

III

Abnormal Nail Colour – red

Erythronychia (red nails)

I Red lunulae – generalized indicates AA along with pitting **AKA 20 nails dystrophy** as it affects all nails

II Localized redness single digit – glomus tumour, subungual cysts or haematomas

III Longitudinal erythronychia (red streak)

Isolated defined ridge in NB corresponds to groove on under-surface of NP due to NM defect ends at the free edge.

A strip where NB is less compressed by overlying nail so that B pools & is more apparent through the thin NP – distally at the free edge - the NP breaks down and the NB will protrude along with a subungual keratosis. assoc with **Dariers disease**

III-defined in the NB which changes with time – due to local glomus tumour or haematoma – may start as a dot and elongate

IV Splinter haemorrhages (red dots/lines on the NB)
trauma
systemic disease – emboli from heart valves

Note the nails may appear a purple red in central cyanosis accompanied by clubbing

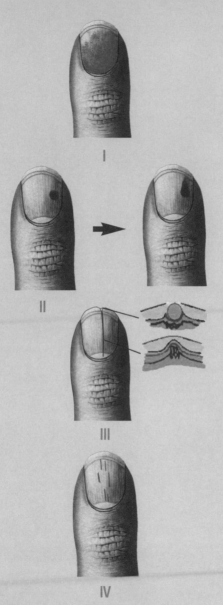

I

II →

III

IV

© A. L. Neill

Abnormal Nail Colour – white

Leukonychia (White/pale nails)

I Apparent leukonychia, pale nails due to the pale NB, assoc anaemia, ß blockers, digital ischaemia **the whiteness disappears on P – to show the pink underneath**

II Isolated leukonychia – due to: a local metaplasia below the NP parakeratois = persistence of nucleated onychocytes subungal filamentous tumour

Muehrcke's paired white bands: bands parallel to lunula with pink in b/w, assoc with hypoalbuminaemia (reversible)

Neopolitan nails: old age; bands of white, brown + red

Pseudoleukonychia is a superficial external whiteness due to onychomycosis – assoc dyshidrosis

III Punctate: 1-3mm pits, minor NM trauma (e.g. manicure)

IV Subtotal leukonychia = white nails with a pink arc 2–4 mm in width distal to the white area. late maturing cells stay white until de-nucleated then become pink. e.g. **Terry's nail:** IVt proximal NP only white - cirrhosis, CCF, DM

Total leukonychia: rare; assoc deafness + epidermal cysts

Transverse = Mees' lines: indicates systemic disease, arsenic poisoning analogous +/- to Beau's lines

V True leukonychia = white discoloration due to NM dysfunction as in onycholysis & parakeratosis – local changes but also assoc. with: AA, carcinoid tumours of the respiratory system, cytotoxic drugs, renal failure, trauma, ulcerative colitis, zinc deficiency. **P on the nail will not change its colour**

VI ½ & ½ nails: proximal is white, sharp demarcation & brownish distally b/n 20-60%; renal failure, uraemia & chemoTx

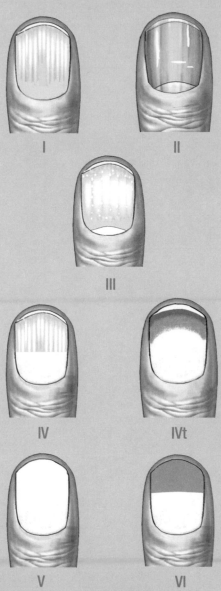

I

II

III

IV

IVt

V

VI

Notes

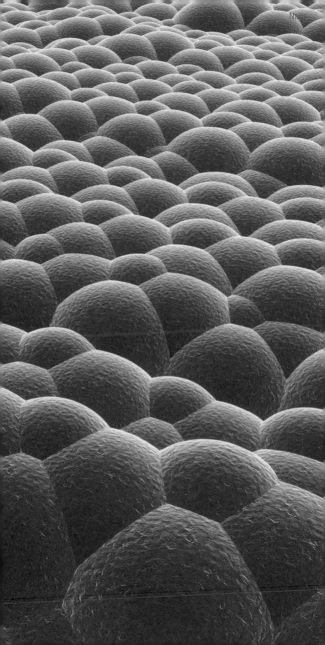

Skin Aging – overview

Skin is b/n 15-25% of the average adult's total weight & covers 50-65 m². The total surface area can change with weight change. Like all CTs it is continually changing & remodeling but this slows with time.

The different layers of the skin show varying changes with time.

1 The Epidermis – thins – comprising of less layers from Sb to Sc, & smaller less adherent cells, which have a reduced turnover cycle. After initially ↑ from birth & childhood, there is estimated to be a 10% loss in the number of keratinocytes per decade after 30yo. Hence the epidermis becomes weaker, dryer & less effective as a barrier to the outside. The epidermal appendages also tend to ↓ in number & size. Hair thins, sweat glands ↓, sebaceous glands become more cellular but secrete less sebum, nails tend to slow in growth rate. The specialized cells of the epidermis also ↓ which has the benefit generally of ↓ atopy, other hypersensitivities & allergies. Melanocytes and other neural crest derived specialized cells cannot reproduce to replace their loss & ↓ with age as do the number of specialized sensory N endings e.g. the Merkel cells, hence reducing the colour & sensitivity of the skin.

2 Dermal-Epidermal Junction – this serrated layer becomes shallower – ↓ the surface area & contact with the Du. Poorer nutrition results in further slowing of the epidermal turnover & ↓ keratinocyte health.

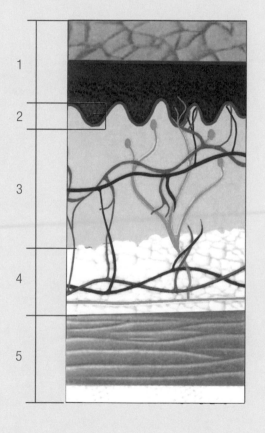

1

2

3

4

5

Skin Aging – overview

3 Dermis – loses both cellular & fibrillar content. It also dehydrates from ⬆ fluid loss, hence it is thinner, dryer, looser & more fragile. The reduction of the specialized epidermal structures further destroy the dermal integrity – with men this is often slowed as they have more coarse terminal hairs particularly on the face.

4 Subcutaneous Tissue – may ⬆ in thickness with age, depending upon the weight of the person. However with dieting and other gross weight changes; the distribution of the fat in this layer fluctuates & generally ends up thinner The face is sensitive to loss in this area due to the ⬆ muscle activity from the muscles of facial expression, forming more defined lines in the skin. Weight gain does not necessarily increase fat in this area.

5 Muscle & Bone mass – below the skin often ⬇ with age further reducing the support base of the skin. In the face this is seen in the malar, mandibular, maxilla regions particularly in those with fewer teeth.

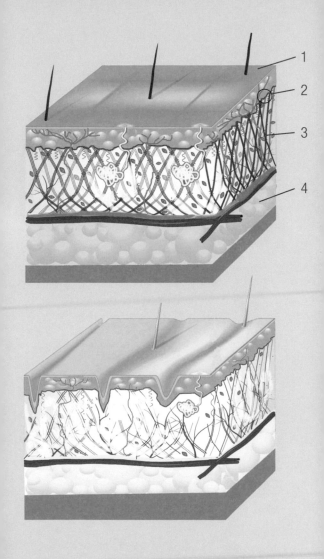

Skin Pigmentation

The main pigment of the skin is MELANIN, synthesized in melanocytes and transferred by "pigment donation", to the keratinocytes. The keratinocytes phagocytose the tips of the melanocytes containing the membrane bound melanin AKA melanosomes.

Darker skin (D) degrades melanin at a slower rate than lighter skins (L), which means there is more melanin and it persists through more of the maturing layers of the epidermis, in dark skins.

The number of melanocytes and the amount of melanin secreted is similar in all skins. There are approximately 35 keratinocytes to each melanocyte. These cells make up ~ 5% of the epidermis.

1 melanocytes
2 premelanosomes formed by the GA
3 melanosomes containing mature melanin phagocytosed by keratinocyte
4 macroautophagy process of melanin degradation in the keratinocyte as it matures - L > D
5 reduction of melanin in L - persistence in D

There are 2 main types of melanin: red yellow melanin - PHAEOMELANIN & the black brown melanin EUMELANIN. The amount of each is genetically determined, and reflected in the colour of the hair, where it is more concentrated.

UV light stimulates the production of both.

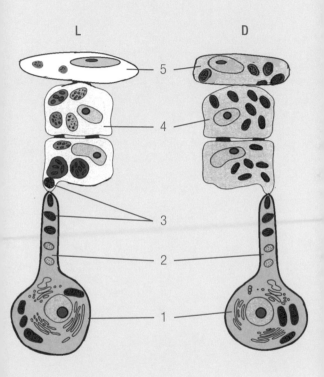

L · · · D

5

4

3

2

1

Skin Tension Lines (STL) / Wrinkles and Photo-aging, RSTLs

STLs are the result of a complex interaction b/n the supf facial muscles of expression & loosening of the attachments of the skin surface to the underlying fat, along with the effects of photo-aging. DSTLs – dynamic skin tension lines - are the result of repeated movements on the face. RSTLs – resting / relaxed skin tension lines – are the result of skin movement & other factors.

DTLs & the Muscles of facial Expression These superficial muscles lie in the subcutaneous fat of the face forming their own fascial plane & acting directly on the skin. Constant movement of these muscles causes STLs - both dynamic = DSTLs - those present in facial movement - & resting (AKA relaxed) = RSTLs present all the time. Both ⬆ with age, & are reinforced by the skin slippage of gravity, when they are called wrinkles or facial lines, & they are generally perpendicular to the movement of the muscles. They are all innervated by CN VII the Facial N. Different anatomic areas of the face have synergistic & antagonist groups of muscles which enable individuals to make varied facial expressions, & form the complex sounds of speech.

Muscles affecting the forehead and eyebrow include:

1 **Frontalis muscle**, which creates the horizontal wrinkles on the forehead & assists with eyebrow elevation

2 **the Corrugators Depressors & Procerus muscles**, which are antagonist to Frontalis & create the wrinkles in the Glabella b/n the eyebrows

3 **the Orbicularis Oculi muscles** shut the eyes & are responsible for the "crows feet" & horizontal lines coming from the lateral canthus of the eyes

4 **Nasalis** this muscle group acts on the nose

5 **the Orbicularis Oris muscles** acts on the mouth & lips used to pronounce the letters M, V, F, & P causing the small longitudinal lines around the lips

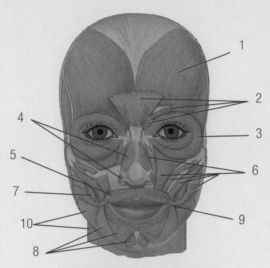

Muscles of facial expression

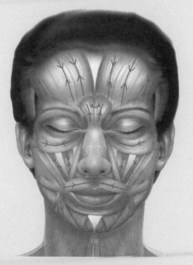

with movements

Skin Tension Lines (STL) / Wrinkles and Photo-aging, RSTLs

6 the Quadratus labii superioris muscles – a group of 6 muscles which act on the upper lip causing the nasolabial fold

7 Buccinator – which assists maintaining the cheek shape - & as the whistling muscle also causes the lip lines

8 the Lip Depressors – a group of 3 muscles which cause the chin DSTLs and the down-turning of the corner of the mouth along with...

9 the mass of the CT **Modiolus** where nearly all the oral muscles insert

10 the Platysma defines the line of the neck and as it ages and elongates – the line softens & becomes pendulous, coursing inferiorly to insert on the skin covering the chin; the mentalis muscle elevates and wrinkles the chin and assists in protruding the lower lip

Further descriptions of muscles in this region are in the A to Z of the Head & Neck Bones & Muscles

RSTLS & Photo-aging (aging from exposure to the sun or UV rays)
Collagen & the other skin fibres are constantly re-modeling – this is altered by exposure to UV radiation – forming aberrant X-links & accelerating the collagen breakdown by up-regulating the normal breakdown enzymes – *metalloproteinases* & ⬆ the aging process. The dermal collagen & elastin fibre based lumps affect the epidermis which is also directly affected by the UV rays resulting in scarred raised keratotic lesions – **actinic keratoses**. This alters **the dermal lines** & loosens & ⬇ the depth of the DE papillae, allowing skin slippage – moving the skin downwards. This occurs in all areas of the body but is generally most evident in the face.

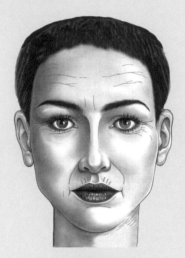

DSTLs

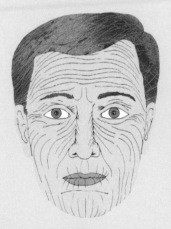

RSTLs

Skin Volume loss / Wrinkles – Face

The face is characteristically divided into 3 sections **the UPPER FACE (UF), the MIDFACE (MF) & the LOWER FACE (LF).** Changes that start early become more pronounced but how the face looks as it ages is multifactoral. These regional changes discussed are added to the general changes of skin as it ages.

The UF main changes with age are: Brow muscle ⬆ (1) prominence & descent; Eye ⬆ STLs (2), Forehead DSTLs become more permanent (3) ➡ to become permanent RSTLs (wrinkles), Glabella b/n the eyes ⬆ DSTLs – wrinkles ⬆(4), Temporal subcutaneous fat & bone thinning – (volume loss) (5).

The MF main changes with age are: Maxilla bone resorption & Malar fat pad drop & medial movement (6) creating volume loss beneath the eyes & in the lateral cheeks, (7) & ⬆ in the Nasolabial fold ⬆(8), also creating lower eyelid drop (9).

The LF main changes with age are: Mandibular bone resorption, elongation of facial muscles with reduced recoil, subcutaneous fat loss & skin droop (gravity), leading to jawline softening (10), jowl and labiomandibular line formation (RSTLs) (11) & double-chin development, and modiolus droop (12) – turning down of the corner of the mouth; ⬆ length of the upper lip leading to ⬆thinning of the lips (13) & ⬆ mental RSTLs b/n chin & lips and chin (14) & neck (15).

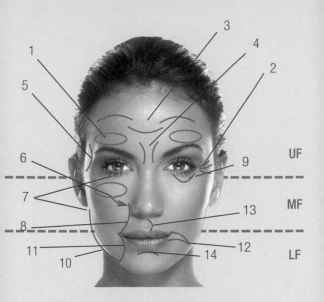

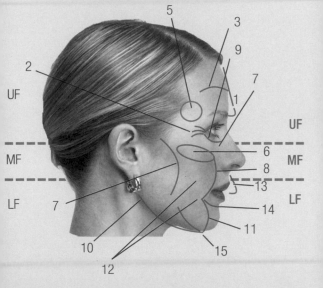

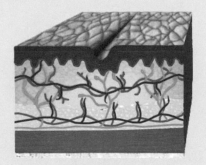

Wrinkle formation

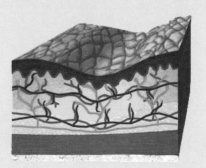

Volume loss

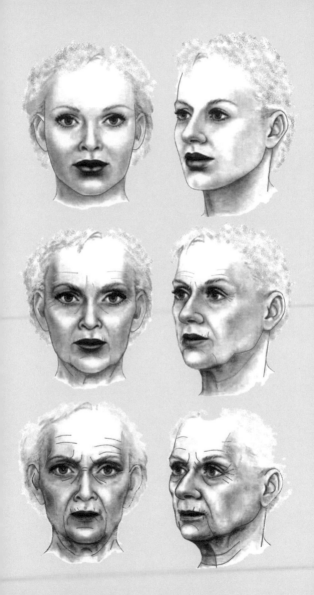

Skin Regional Differences – (relative scale 0-6)

		FACE general	FACE	FACE
	Axilla / Anogenital	Face	Lip – vermillion border	Nose
Sc thickness	2	2	0	2
E thickness	2	2	1	2
BM	1	1	1	2
DE	2	2	1	3
collagen bands	2	3	1	3
sweat glands	4	4	0	1
sebaceous glands	4	4 ♂ > ♀	0	6 ♂ > ♀
Dermal thickness	1	3	3	2
HF density ↓ with age	4	4 ♂ > ♀	0	3 ♂ > ♀
presence of skel mu	0	6	6	6
subcut fat thickness	2	3-6	1	1

Back	Forearm	Abdomen	Scalp	Solar / Volar surfaces
2	2	2	3	6
2	2	2	2	6
4	2	2	2	6
3	2	2	3	6
6	3	2	2	5
3	2	2	4	6
2	2	1	4	0
6	3	2	3	6
2 ♂ > ♀	2 ♂ > ♀	2	4 ♂ > ♀ with age	0
0	0	0	0-4	4
3-6	2-5	3-6 or more	2	2-4

Skin Types

When assessing skin for risk of melanoma it is often helpful to "type" its potential for sun damage. The most used form of typing is the FITZPATRICK SCALE.

The Fitzpatrick Scale - of skin type

Skin Type	Skin Colour	Sun reaction to skin	Other Associated features
I	White or freckled skin	**Always burns, never tans**	light / blue coloured eyes light hair
II	White skin	**Burns easily, tans poorly**	light to medium eye colour light to medium hair colour
III	Olive skin	**Mild burn, gradually tans**	brown eyes brown hair
IV	Light brown skin	**Burns minimally, tans easily**	brown / black hair brown / black eyes
V	Dark brown skin	**Rarely burns, tans easily**	black curly / kinky hair brown / black eyes
VI	Black skin	**Never burns, always tans**	black, kinky hair brown / black eyes

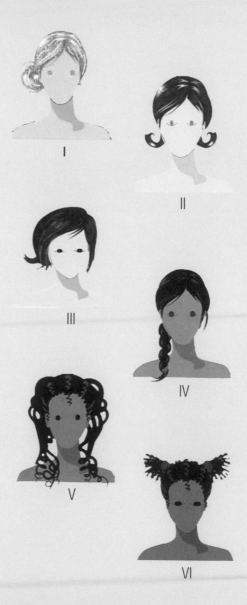

I

II

III

IV

V

VI

Blood Supply & Lymphatic drainage of the Skin

The skin's BVs arise from underlying **source vessels**, which are terminal branches of muscular BVs or direct perforating BVs. Each of the BVs supply a region from the skin to the bone – an angiosome & connect with adjacent angiosomes via reduced calibre (choke) vessels or similar caliber (true) anastomotic vessels, so the BF to whole areas can be controlled.

BVs travel in the CT, fascial plane & supply branches to the surrounding Ts. The arteries emerge from the deep fascia in the muscular septa or near the tendons & travel through the subcutaneous T (Su) toward the skin. In the dermis (D) they form extensive horizontal subdermal = deep & dermal = superficial plexi, which are connected via communicating vessels oriented perpendicular to the skin surface. The upper BVs all anastomose to form a **continuous vascular network w / in the skin**, specifically protruding into the dermal papillae. Clinically, this extensive horizontal BV network is the reason the avascular epidermis (E) is able to heal so rapidly.

Lymphatics follow the BVs beginning as open – ended channels in the dermal papillae; with ⬆ BF there is ⬆ fluid in the T – w / o lymphatics the skin can stretch and swell up to 5X causing lymphoedema.

1 **dermal papillae & capillaries**

2 **superficial dermal plexus / continuous vascular network**

3 **supf communicating BVs**

4 **deep dermal plexus**

5 **deep communicating BVs**

6 **source vessels**

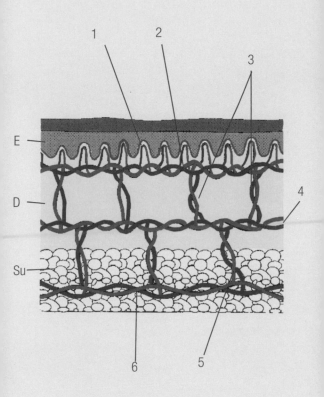

E

D

Su

Thermoregulation – via BVs of the skin

Heat is lost from the skin via sweat glands, convection & directed BF. There are 20X more capillaries in the skin than necessary so generally only 5% of the capillary beds are open at any one time, but via the SyNS, constriction & dilatation of cutaneous BVs can be altered, to lose more or less heat. Note lack of oxygen will override these central controls.

1 terminal arteriole
2 metarteriole
3 precapillary sphincter c = closed / o = open
4 capillaries ⬇ when the bed is isolated
5 thoroughfare – capillary bed bypass
6 venuole
7 smooth muscle of the BV art > ven
8 capillary bed
9 Sym N on the arteriole sphincters & arterioles

Glomus bodies are specialized local capillary beds found in the skin. More "knotted" than normal capillary beds, they can push a lot of B through quickly when open, but can almost completely shut down, changing their size considerably. They are found in / near the dermal papillae as close to the surface as possible, concentrated in the fingertips.

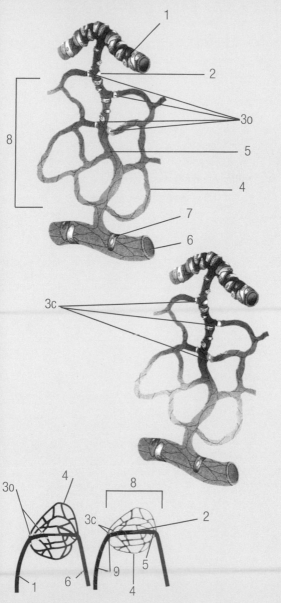

Dermis – overview

The primary function of the D is to sustain & support the epidermis. It has 2 layers, **the upper dermis (Du) = the superficial papillary dermis & the deep dermis (Dd) = the reticular dermis.**

The Dd is a thick layer of dense CT, with closely interlaced elastic fibres 1% & coarse bundles of collagen fibres 70% arranged parallel to the surface, & in defined tracts called **Dermal lines**. Cutting along them rather than across them ⬇ healing time & scarring. The other T components of the Dd are irregular & border the subcutaneous T layer = the panniculus adiposus, which lies on the deep fascial layer of the body.

The Du is thinner, consisting of loose CT containing: capillaries (1), collagen (2), elastic (3) & reticular fibres (4) & lymphatics (5).

The gel-like ground substance of the D 29% is composed of mucopolysaccharides (primarily hyaluronic acid), chondroitin sulphates, & glycoprotein & is responsible for the skin's turgor. It supports the epidermal appendages.

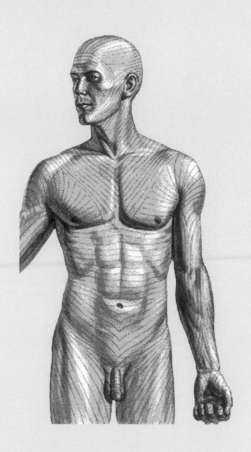

Dermis – microanatomy

Resident dermal cells include: adipocytes = fat cells (6) , fibroblasts (7b), fibrocytes (7c), histiocytes (8), lymphocytes (9), mast cells (10), macrophages (11), plasma cells (12) & the rare polymorphonuclear cell (13). It is loose CT = areolar T; thicker and stiffer in males than females, supporting more glands, hair & containing more collagen fibres.

Fibroblasts / Fibrocytes, Elastin & Collagen The fibrocyte is the major cell types of the dermis. It produces & secretes pro-collagen & elastic fibers. Pro-collagen is extruded from the cell, then cleaved by extracellular enzymes & it aggregates with X-linking to form collagen or add to the existing collagen fibres. Collagen fibres are strong, helical fibrils rotating around each other in increasing sizes. They provide the skin's tensile strength & R to shear & other mechanical forces. The elastic fibers are much less in number but play an enormous functional role by returning the skin to its resting shape after deformation. Fibrocytes and hence the fibres ⬇ with age accounting for ⬆ skin tears & fragility of skin, & ⬆ skin sagging.

Mast cells / Histiocytes = Resident Macrophages These are the immune cells of the D. **Mast cells** are **basophils** which moved out from the BS. They "explode" when triggered by an Ag (which may come from the epidermal Langerhan cells) releasing their granules into the ground substance causing severe acute hypersensitivity reactions – as in allergies. Monocytes also leave the BS & reside in the T – **Histiocytes = Resident macrophages** they "mop up" the debris in this area via phagocytosis. They can undergo epitheloid & other changes in response to T injury & invasion.

Dermo-epidermal junction The **dermo-epidermal junction (DE)** is an undulating BM that adheres the E to the D. It is composed of 2 layers, the **lamina lucida & lamina densa**. The **lamina lucida** is thinner & lies directly beneath the basal layer of epidermal keratinocytes. Hemidesmosomes stick the cells of the Sb onto this layer. **The thicker lamina densa** is in direct contact with the underlying D. Dermal papillae from the Du contain a plexus of capillaries & lymphatics oriented perpendicular to the skin surface. These fingerlike projections are surrounded by similar projections of the epidermis -the rete ridges. This highly irregular junction greatly increases the surface area over which oxygen, nutrients, & waste products are exchanged b/n the dermis & the avascular epidermis, and protects the skin from excessive frictional forces. The epidermal appendages: glands & hair invaginate at the base of the DP taking epithelial cells & BM with them & enclose them as they descend deeply into the D.

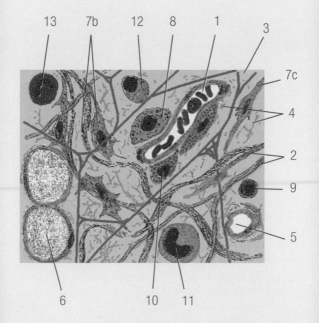

Epidermal appendages (EA)

These are defined as structures which are of epithelial origin. They are connected to the E but may lie in the D - intradermal epithelial structures lined with epithelial cells. These are an important store of epithelial cells, which may be the source of re-epithelialization should the overlying E be removed or destroyed e.g. in abrasions, burns & iatrogenially in skin graft harvesting.

EA include the following:

Hair (although this has both E & D components) – see separate HAIR section; Glands: apocrine eccrine, mammary & sebaceous; & Nails – see separate NAIL section.

1 **Apocrine glands** Apocrine glands develop at puberty & are assoc. with HF in the axillae, the anogenital region. Modified apocrine glands are also in the external ear canal (ceruminous glands), the eyelid (Moll's glands) & the breast (mammary glands). They are odoriferous, and probably have a vestigial function – of sexual attraction, pheromone production.

2 **Sebaceous glands** are holocrine glands directly assoc. with HFs and found in all areas of hairy skin. They are largest & densest in the face & scalp where they are the sites of origin of acne. They produce & secrete sebum, a group of complex oils including: triglycerides, fatty acids, wax esters, squalene & cholesterol and their own cell debris. Sebum lubricates the skin (& hair) acting as a barrier to bacteria, water, frictional & shearing forces. It is slightly acidic pH (5.5-6.5).

3 **Sweat glands** are eccrine glands found over the entire surface of the body (2-3 million /body) except the vermillion border of the lips, the external ear canal, the NBs, the labia minora & the glans penis. They are most concentrated in the axilla, palms & soles. The coiled secretory intradermal portion (manufactures the sweat – NaCl) is connected to the E via a relatively straight distal duct (which concentrates it). They produce sweat to cool the body by evaporation. The thermoregulatory center in the hypothalamus controls sweat gland activity through the SyNS. Sweat excretion is triggered when core body temperature reaches or exceeds a set point.

See also Terms and Definitions section for further discussion.

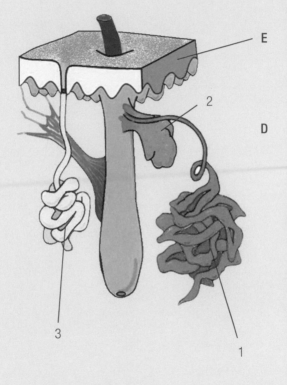

E

2

D

3

1

Epidermis - layers, cells & barriers

The epidermis does not contain BVs relying on **the dermis** for nutrient delivery & waste disposal via diffusion through **the dermoepidermal junction**.

The epidermis is a stratified, squamous epithelium consisting of keratinocytes in progressive stages of differentiation from deeper to more superficial layers.

The named layers of the epidermis include

1 the stratum basale (Sb),

2 stratum spinosum (Ss),

3 stratum granulosum (Sg),

4 stratum lucidum (SL), &

5 stratum corneum (Sc).

Cell types which exist in the epidermis are **keratinocyes (6)**, which can only divide in the Sb(8), **Antigen presenting cells AKA Langerhans cells (9)** found in all the epidermal layers; **Melanocytes AKA Pigment producing cells (10)** which supply the keratinocytes with pigment ~1:34 cells. This decreases with age so the person is paler, and more vulnerable to skin diseases, and **the Sensory cells AKA Merkel cells (11)**, which respond to light touch.

As the epidermal layers progress to the surface they release proteins and lipids to act as a water proof barrier for the skin. The barrier prevents the skin drying out as well as protecting the skin from external invasion.

12 hemidesmosome (h)- attachment of Sb epithelial cells to the BM & Ds (d)- strong intercellular connection, Sb, Ss loosening in the SL & Sc

13 keratin granules, Sg, SL, Sc

14 LBs - release lipids & proteins into the SL

15 protein & lipid barrier, SL

16 keratin fibres filling the cells, Sc & corneocytes flaking off

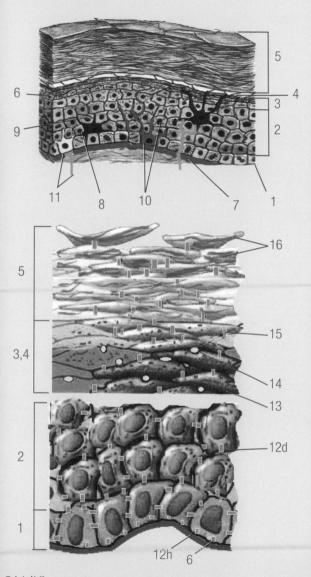

Epidermis – cell types

Keratinocytes The Sb is attached to the **basement membrane (BM)** via **hemidesmosomes** & to each other via desmosomes – specialized areas for intercellular communication. It is the only layer capable of cell division = **mitosis**. The upper layer of dead keratinocytes, the Sc, is the largest & varies in thickness b/n 3-5mm in the eyelid to >150mm in the volar & solar surfaces. Cells are shed daily and replaced by those below. Excessive production of keratinocytes particularly in the Sc = **keratosis** results in a number of pathological skin conditions

The Merkel cell (Mc) Merkel cells are derived from neural crest cells – and act as extensions of N processes. They are specialized sensory receptors for light touch, lie in the base of the dermal papillae and are concentrated in highly sensitive areas – finger tips, nail beds & genitalia. Their base is attached to sensory Ns, through the BM. They detect small changes in the P of the keratinocytes (E) via intercellular communications – desmosomes (Ds) which feed into the N cell (N) via granules (G) so generating a N impulse.

1 **corneocyte**
2 **granulocyte**
3 **spinocyte**
4 **basal cell**
5 **desmosone**
6 **hemidesmosone**
7 **BM**
8 **Merkel cell**
9 **N cell process**

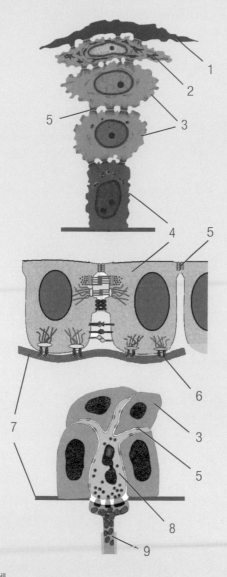

Map of Sensory Innervation of the Skin - Dermatomes & Peripheral Nerves

Most of the body's sensory perception comes through the skin. Overlapping sections of the skin are supplied by individual Spinal Nerves called Dermatomes.

Peripheral Nerves are made up of a number of Spinal Nerves which may contribute to several Peripheral Nerves, the areas of the skin they receive sensory input is different to that of the Dermatomes. The Trigeminal Nerve - or 5th Cranial Nerve - has 3 parts which supply 3 sections of the face.

ANTERIOR
DERMATOMES
(SEGMENTAL) - cutaneous distribution of the N roots

PERIPHERAL NERVES

1 Greater Auricular N
2 Supraclavicular Ns + Anterior cutaneous N of the neck
3 Intercostal Ns anterior + lateral branches
4 Axillary N
5 Medial cutaneous N of the arm + forearm (brachial + antebrachial)
6 Inferior lateral cutaneous branches of the Radial N
7 Musculocutaneous N
8 Median N
9 Ulnar N
10 Iliohypogastric + Genitofemoral N
11 Ilioinguinal + Genitofemoral N
12 Lateral Femoral cutaneous N
13 Obturator N
14 Femoral N (ant. cut. branch)
15 Saphenous branch of Femoral N
16 Superficial Peroneal N
17 Deep Peroneal N
18 Tibial N
19 Greater Occipital N
20 Cutaneous branches of the Dorsal rami
21 Trigeminal N / ganglion
21i Ophthalmic N
21ii Maxillary N
21iii Mandibular N

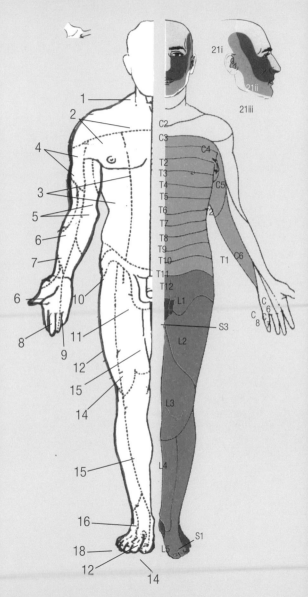

21i

21ii

21iii

1

2

C2

C3

4

C4

T2

3

T3

T4

C5

5

T5

6

T6

T2

7

T7

T8

T9

6

T10

T1

C6

10

T11

T12

8

L1

9

S3

11

L2

12

C6

15

C8 C7

14

L3

15

L4

16

S1

18

L5

12

14

© A. L. Neill

227

Map of Sensory Innervation of the Skin - Dermatomes & Peripheral Nerves

POSTERIOR
DERMATOMES
(SEGMENTAL - cutaneous distribution of the N roots)

PERIPHERAL NERVES

1   Greater Auricular N
2   Supraclavicular Ns + Anterior cutaneous N of the neck
3   Intercostal Ns anterior + lateral branches
4   Axillary N
5   Medial Cutaneous N of the arm +forearm (brachial + antebrachial)
6   Inferior lateral cutaneous branches of the Radial N
7   Musculocutaneous N
8   Median N
9   Ulnar N
10 Iliohypogastric + Genitofemoral N
11 Ilioinguinal + Genitofemoral N
12 Lateral Femoral cutaneous N
13 Obturator N
14 Femoral N (ant. cut. branch)
15 Saphenous branch of Femoral N
16 Superficial Peroneal N
17 Deep Peroneal N
18 Tibial N
19 Greater Occipital N
20 Cutaneous branches of the Dorsal rami

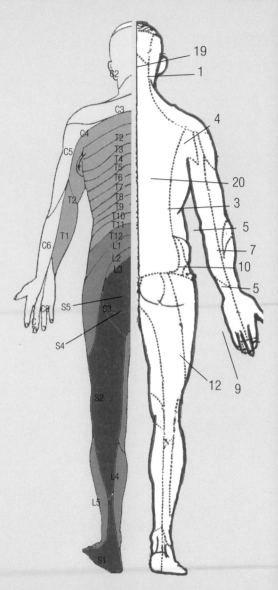

Map of Sensory Innervation of the Skin of the Head and Neck

The Face is innervated by the Trigeminal N = CN V & its branches.
The top of the head and neck by the upper cervical spinal Ns

1 Supra-orbital N (V_1)

2 Supratrochlear N (V_1)

3 Lacrimal N (V_1)

4 Infratrochlear N (V_1)

5 External nasal N (V_1)

6 Zygomaticofacial N (V_2)

7 Infra-orbital N (V_2)

8 Mental N (V_3)

9 Buccal N (V_3)

10 Great Auricular N (C2,3)

11 anterior cutaneous N of the Neck (C2-3)

12 dorsal branches of C6

13 dorsal branches of C5

14 dorsal branches of C4

15 dorsal branches of C3

16 Auriculotemporal N (V_2)

17 Lesser Occipital N (C1,2)

18 Greater Occipital N (C2)

19 Zygomaticotemporal N (V_2)

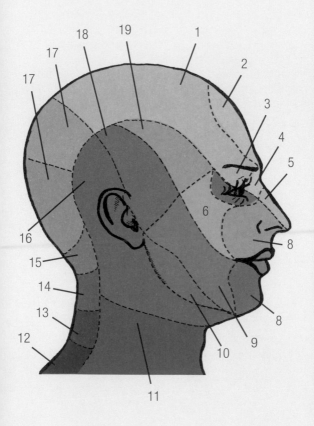

Skin Afferent Nerves – Ending Specializations

The Skin is responsible for most tactile detection via mechanical changes to its surface using at least 5 morphologically distinct afferent N endings, which have specialized sensitivities – T position, pressure & other mechanical changes = mechanoreceptors. As well as the shape differences – other differences found w/n & across these different N ending types are: the size of the receptive field, the rate of reaction & the adaptability. Other modalities detected in the skin include:

temperature changes – thermoreceptors – mild temperature changes - Free N endings, cold receptors – Bulboid (Krause N endings) **pain – nociceptors**, Free N endings*

Bulboid corpuscles = end-bulbs of Krause – thermoceptors & mechanoreceptors *detect* low-frequency vibration, P, cold temperatures. *morphology* They are minute CT encapsulated soft, semi-fluid oval bodies, in which the N fibre terminates in a coiled-up plexiform mass. *location* the conjunctiva of the eye, MMs of the lips & tongue, distal finger jts, the penis & clitoris

Bulbous corpuscles = Ruffini corpuscles – slowly adapting mechanoreceptors *detect* – skin stretching, slippage & deep P – modulating finger grip strength & type, heat *morphology* – long cylindrical capsule filled with free N endings *location* – the dermal layers, & w/n joints, proprioceptive

* although if "overstimulated" all receptors will report pain

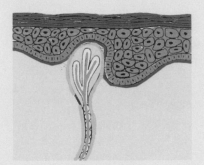

Bulbous – Krause

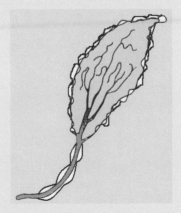

Bulbous – Ruffini

Skin Afferent Nerves – Ending Specializations

Lamella = Pacinian corpuscles – rapidly adapting mechanoreceptors – with a wide receptor field *detect* – rapid vibrations partic b/n 100-300 Hz, gross P changes, but not constant P

morphology – large – 1 X 1mm knobs which contain free N endings wrapped in modified Schwann cell coverings 60-100 thin CT concentric laminae with gelatinous coverings and swimming in fluid

location – sparsely located throughout the deep dermis

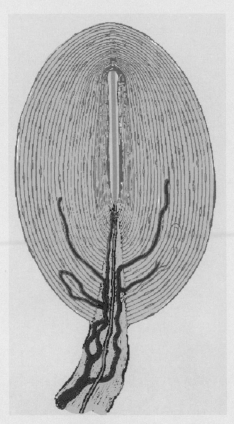

Pacinian corpuscles

Skin Afferent Nerves – Ending Specializations

Merkel cell neurite complex = slowly adapting mechanoreceptors *detect* sustained touch & pressure, and very low vibration up to 10Hz, sensitive finger tip texture detection & pattern changes & 2 point discrimination *morphology* free N ending closely assoc. with a Merkel cell – which is in the SBasale of the skin *location* a wide distribution of the supf skin layers at the base of the dermal papillae. In particular these cells are concentrated around the hair unit in collected "touch domes" / hair discs, in the nipple region, in the MM of the mouth and anus & at the base finger tip dermal papillae.

Tactile = Meissner's corpuscles - rapidly adapting mechanoreceptors – with a small receptor field & low activation threshold *detect* light touch, low vibrations 50Hz, texture changes *morphology* medium sized 70 X 80µm knobs which contain free N endings covered in modified Schwann cell coverings up to 20 layers *location* concentrated in areas especially sensitive to light touch: the finger tips, the lips & w/n the dermal papillae of the skin – note the numbers ⬇ to 25% by 50yo – this may be due to their very supf location – not found in hairy skin

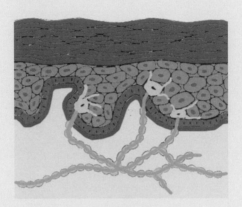

Merkel

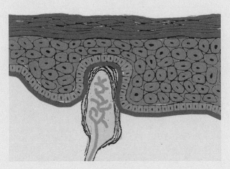

Meissner

Skin Afferent Nerves – Ending Specializations

Free N endings = nociceptors + Hair afferent fibres *detect* light touch, movement of HS, pain *morphology* free un-myelinated ends *location* found around the HF to the top of the bulbar region, noting the change in hair angle, also found loose in the skin T deep & supf. layers.

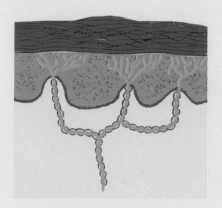

Free N endings

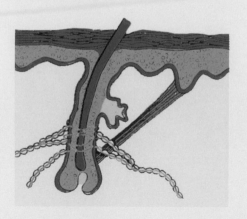

Phases of Wound Healing – overview

The entire wound healing process is a complex series of events that begins at the moment of injury & can continue for months to years.

There are 3 main phases to this process.

I Inflammatory Phase Immediate to 2-5 days

Haemostasis
Vasoconstriction
Platelet aggregation
Thromboplastin forms the clot
Inflammation
Vasodilation – reperfusion
Phagocytosis – of debris

1 defect – ulcer in the skin
2 cut BV – bleeding, then constricted so bleeding stops
3 fibrin , platelets
4 clot
5 constricted BV

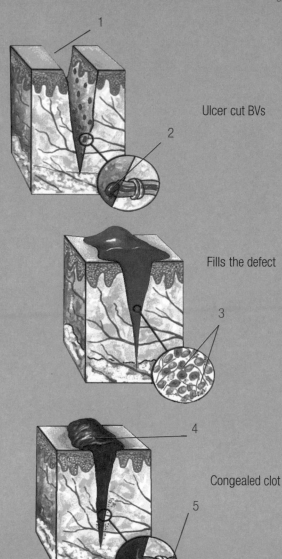

Ulcer cut BVs

Fills the defect

Congealed clot

© A. L. Neill

Phases of Wound Healing – overview

The entire wound healing process is a complex series of events that begins at the moment of injury & can continue for months to years.

II Proliferative Phase 2 days to 3 weeks

Granulation Fibroblasts lay bed of collagen
the defect fills with serum & produces new capillaries
Contraction Wound edges pull together to reduce defect size
Re-epithelialization Crosses moist surface – and if the ulcer is extensive comes from the epithelium of the epidermal appendages. An epithelial cell can travel about 3 cm from point of origin in all directions.

III Remodeling Phase 3 weeks to 2 years

New collagen forms which ↑ tensile strength to wounds – & continues to re-model Scar tissue is at its maximum 80% as strong as original tissue

1. scab
2. exudate
3. granulation T
4. ↑ BVs
5. cell types fibrocytes, lymphocytes, macrophages
6. new migratory epithelial cells

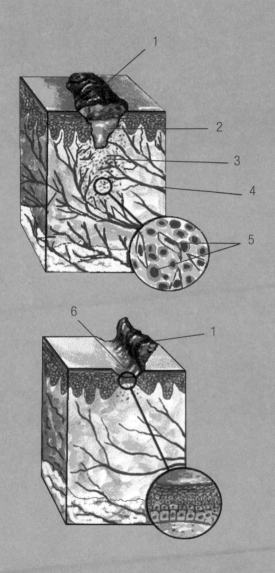

HOW TO DESCRIBE SKIN LESIONS

It is important to know how to describe a skin lesion in a systematic easy to understand manner

1. SITE (S)

2. SIZE (S) - average or range & variability of each –

3. ERYTHEMATOUS or NOT - red or not - hot or not

4. DURATION - acute < 2 weeks / chronic > 2weeks

5. SURFACE FEATURES
   Normal / Smooth – i.e. the same as the surrounding skin
   Crusty – with ulcer
   Excoriated – injured
   Exudates / erosions
   Hairy - ectopically
   Horny / keratin thickened
   Scaly / increased skin production
   Warty / Papillomatous

6. FLAT – macules or patches (determined by size) or
   RAISED – papules, vesicles, & pustules or plaques,
   nodules & bullae

7. NON-BLANCHABLE COLOUR
   skin-coloured, or pink, red, mauve, purple, brown, white,
   yellow, cream or golden

© A. L. Neill

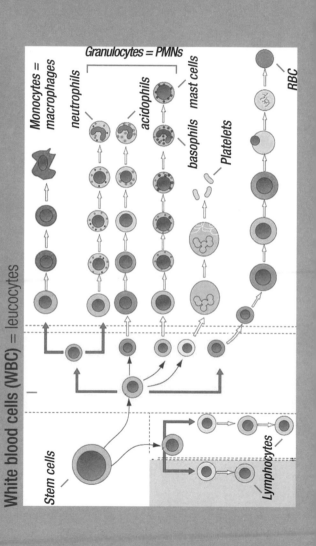

White blood cells (WBC) = leucocytes

Monocytes = macrophages

Granulocytes = PMNs

neutrophils

acidophils

mast cells

basophils

Platelets

RBC

Stem cells

Lymphocytes